CARDIOVASCULAR DISEASES

OXFORD MONOGRAPHS ON MEDICAL GENETICS

General Editors

ARNO G. MOTULSKY   MARTIN BOBROW
PETER S. HARPER   CHARLES SCRIVER

Former Editors

J.A. FRASER ROBERTS   C.O. CARTER

OXFORD MONOGRAPHS ON MEDICAL GENETICS NO. 22

CARDIOVASCULAR DISEASES
Genetics, Epidemiology, and Prevention

James J. Nora, MD, MPH
University of Colorado School of Medicine

Kåre Berg, MD
University of Oslo

Audrey Hart Nora, MD, MPH
United States Public Health Service

New York   Oxford
OXFORD UNIVERSITY PRESS
1991

Oxford University Press

Oxford   New York   Toronto
Delhi   Bombay   Calcutta   Madras   Karachi
Petaling Jaya   Singapore   Hong Kong   Tokyo
Nairobi   Dar es Salaam   Cape Town
Melbourne   Auckland

and associated companies in
Berlin   Ibadan

Copyright © 1991 by James J. Nora, Kåre Berg, Audrey Hart Nora

Published by Oxford University Press, Inc.,
200 Madison Avenue, New York, New York 10016

Oxford is a registered trademark of Oxford University Press

Library of Congress Cataloging-in-Publication Data

Nora, James J., 1928–
   Cardiovascular diseases : genetics, epidemiology, and prevention /
James J. Nora, Kåre Berg, Audrey Hart Nora.
      p.   cm.—(Oxford monographs on medical genetics ; no. 22)
   Includes bibliographical references and index.
   ISBN 0-19-506032-6 ✓
   1. Congenital heart disease. 2. Heart—Diseases—Genetic aspects.
3. Heart—Diseases—Epidemiology. 4. Heart—Diseases—Prevention.
I. Berg, Kåre. II. Nora, Audrey Hart, 1936–   . III. Title
IV. Series.
   [DNLM: 1. Cardiovascular Diseases—epidemiology.
2. Cardiovascular Diseases—genetics 3. Cardiovascular Diseases—
prevention & control. WG 100 N822c]
RC687.N67 1991   616.1—dc20   DNLM/DLC
for Library of Congress   90-14339

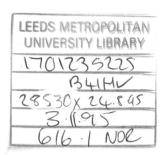
9   8   7   6   5   4   3   2   1

Printed in the United States of America
on acid-free paper

Contents

Introduction

Knowledge of what casues cardiovascular diseases has progressed at a pace that challenges not only the student, but the physician and the research scientist. And while there is scientific merit in discovering the etiology of any disease, the ultimate goal is to apply what we learn to the treatment, and possibly to the prevention, of the diseases being studied. In this volume we propose to bring together what we understand about the causes and prevention of cardiovascular diseases in individuals, families, and societies. Our first theme, variations of which will be played throughout this work, is: cardiovascular diseases are familial.

It is an enjoyable exercise for geneticists to trace the history of the awareness of the familial nature of a disease to its first description, such as Hippocrates suggesting that epilepsy ran in families. For cardiovascular diseases, perhaps Morgagni (1769) should be credited as the first to describe a familial occurrence—apparent strokes in two generations of a family (although the important contributions of hypertension and its genetic basis were not apparent until this century).

Fogge described familial xanthoma (1873) and Sir William Osler (1897), citing the Matthew Arnold family, called attentin to the familial nature of angina pectoris. (Indeed, in 1951, Levine in his widely used textbook, *Clinical Heart Disease,* stated that in angina pectoris: "Probably the most important etiologic factor is heredity.") Müller (1938) recognized the additional feature of familial hypercholesterolemia and the dominant mode of inheritance. With the emergence of epidemiologic studies in the 1960s and 1970s, the role of family history among coronary risk factors was less emphasized. However, genetic factors in early-onset coronary heart disease are currently the focus of research at the forefront of medicine.

The next major category of cardiovascular disease to be appreciated as having a familial aspect was rheumatic fever (Cheadle, 1889). In the 1930s, familial clusters of different cardiovascular diseases were being recognized, but it was Wilson and Schweitzer (1937) who were the first to attempt a formal genetic analysis of one of these disorders. They proposed that susceptibility to rheumatic fever was best explained by inheritance of a single autosomal recessive gene. As early as 1931, Coburn had suggested a streptococcal etiology, but even in the 1950s there were those who were not prepared to embrace this concept. Reviewing the older literature on the genetics of rheumatic fever is a lesson in humility for all of us who try to understand the genetic and environmental contributions to disease. The cornerstone in today's approach to rheumatic fever is the prompt treatment of beta-hemolytic group A streptococcal infections in those who have not had rheumatic fever, and the prevention of subsequent streptococcal infections in those who have had the disease (through lifetime antibiotic prophylaxis). But there is clearly a genetic aspect to rheumatic fever and this will be discussed further in Chapter 3.

Familial dysrhythmias were recognized by Morquio (1901) and Osler (1903). Because dysrhythmia and cardiomyopathy so often occur together, there is a pedagogical reason for combining these disorders in one chapter, as we have done in this presentation, despite the fact that it makes an overly heterogeneous grouping from the point of view of etiology.

Congenital heart disease was the last of the five major categories of cardiovascular disease to attract genetic investigators. Kindreds with more than one individual with a congenital heart disease appeared sporadically in the literature before the first systematic studies were undertaken in the 1950s. These early studies were impeded by the state of the art because there were significant limitations in the knowledge of diagnosis of congenital heart disease in the living patient. Also, methods sometimes employed were unsuited for informative studies of this problem (e.g., mailed questionnaires). Technical advances in other areas have made possible the more revealing etiologic studies from the 1960s to the present day. Explicit in the title of this volume is the recognition by the authors that genetic factors for most cardiovascular diseases interact in important, perhaps critical ways with the environment. Epidemiology and the genetic-environmental interaction are of such consequence in the pathogenesis of the diseases to be discussed here that our title could easily be *Cardiovascular Diseases: Genetic–Epidemiology, and Prevention.* Whether a comma or hyphen is used between genetics and epidemiology, the role of the environment is major, particularly in prevention. Our hope is that the pages that follow will be as useful in stimulating questions as they are in providing a concise resource of current information.

Denver, February 1991	*J.J.N.*
Oslo, February 1991	*K.B.*
Denver, February 1991	*A.H.N.*

REFERENCES

Cheadle, W.B. (1889). Harveian lectures on the various manifestations of the rheumatic state as exemplified in childhood and early life. *Lancet* **I**, 821, 871, 921.

Fogge, C.H. (1873. *Trans. Path. Soc.* **24,** 242.

Morgagni, J.B. (1769). *The Seats and Causes of Disease Investigated by Anatomy.* London.

Morquio, L. (1901). *Arch. Med. Enfants*. **4,** 467.

Müller, C. (1938). *Acta Med. Scand.* (suppl.) **89,** 75.

Osler, W. (1897). *Lectures on Angina Pectoris and Allied States*. D. Appleton & Co., New York.

Osler, W. (1903). *Lancet* **II,** 516.

Wilson, M.G., and Schweitzer, M.D. (1937). *J. Clin. Invest*. **16,** 555.

CARDIOVASCULAR DISEASES

1

Atherosclerosis and Coronary Artery Disease

In many industrialized countries, coronary artery disease (CAD) continues to be the most common cause of death. More than 1,250,000 heart attacks occur every year in the United States and over 500,000 people die every year as a result of this disease. For 20–30% of heart attack victims, the first clue to the presence of the disease is sudden death. CAD reached its peak in the United States in 1963 and remained at that level for the rest of the decade before beginning to decline rather sharply. By 1988 there was a better than one-third reduction in deaths from CAD as compared with 1972. Nevertheless, cardiovascular diseases are still the predominant cause of death in the United States. A promising decline in the frequency of CAD has also been observed in Western European countries. In Norway, for example, there has been a 20% reduction in CAD mortality in men 40–59 years old since the early 1970s.

Since death is inescapable, it is not given that one cause of death is worse than another. It can be argued that a cardiac death is preferable to a cancer death if it occurs in old age following a long and meaningful life. What makes CAD such a serious public health problem is that it so often kills or incapacitates people who are still leading an active professional and private life and whose families may be heavily dependent on them. Despite the recent decline in CAD frequency, the current risk of dying from CAD is 3.5: 1,000 per year for men aged 50–59 years in Western European populations (such as the Norwegian). It is a major challenge to prevent the early cases of CAD and to delay disease development as much as possible in those susceptible to CAD. It is our conviction that the medical geneticists have a major role to play in the efforts to prevent or delay the development of CAD.

Until relatively recently, it was generally assumed that except for rare cases of monogenic hyperlipidemia, genetic factors were of only minor importance in the etiology of CAD. Despite the inertia with respect to genetic factors in CAD, genetic interest in the disorder is over a century old. In the English literature, the first mention of the familial aspect of CAD with xanthomatosis was made by Fogge (1873). Thanks to Sir William Osler (1897) we learned that familial angina, without the emphasis on the sentinel abnormality of familial xanthomatosis, could recur in families and that this was perhaps first appreciated not by a physician, but by a poet and essayist Matthew Arnold. While visiting the United States in 1887, Arnold experienced his first attack of angina pectoris and wrote to a friend: that he began to think that his time was really coming to an end. He had so much pain in his chest, which was the sign of a malady which had suddenly struck in middle life, long before they came to his present age, both his father and his grandfather. Matthew Arnold lived with chest pain for less than a year before he died on April 15, 1888. One of his biographers disclosed amazingly little scholarship when he described the cause of Arnold's death as "heart failure . . . sudden and quite unexpected." Unexpected—except by Matthew Arnold.

In the late 1930s, the Norwegian professor of medicine Carl Müller examined and reported several Norwegian kindreds in which the triad of xanthomatosis, CAD, and hypercholesterolemia segregated as an autosomal dominant trait (Müller, 1939). Since that time, it has been broadly accepted that familial hypercholesterolemia is an autosomal dominant trait. However, for a long while the tacit assumption seemed to be that familial hypercholesterolemia in the etiology of CAD represented a very rare exception in a disorder generally caused by nutritional or lifestyle factors.

In recent years, it has become increasingly clear that the majority of CAD cases are caused by a combination of genetic and environmental factors. Genetic factors apparently are particularly important when CAD occurs at a relatively young age. However, even when it is admitted that genetic factors may play an important role, it is often stated that "there is nothing one can do about genes." This has created the impression that there is little or nothing one can do to prevent disease in people who have genetic risk factors predisposing to CAD. The implausibility of this defeatist attitude is illustrated by the drastic reduction in CAD frequency in several European countries during World War II. This reduction was of such magnitude that many people with a strong genetic predisposition to contract CAD must have escaped disease during the war years.

Whenever environmental as well as genetic factors are of importance in the etiology of a disease, the unifying concept is that the environmental factors preferentially cause disease in people with a genetic predisposition. There is little doubt that the relative contribution of genetic factors and environmental factors differs between cases. For the time being, it may be useful to think in terms of the following broad categories of mechanisms that may be involved in determining CAD risk:

1. Risk exclusively caused by environmental/lifestyle factors (i.e., heavy smoking or excessive fat intake)
2. Risk caused by single genes determining a high risk factor level
3. Gene-environment interaction expressed as
   a. differences between genotypes with respect to risk factor variability (see below), or

b. risk factor and marker gene associations depending on presence or absence of specific environmental factors such as smoking
4. Gene-gene interactions as exemplified by the cholesterol increasing effect of the apolipoprotein E4 (apoE4) allele being eliminated by the presence of a normal gene at the low density lipoprotein receptor (LDLR) locus (see below).

In this chapter, we will summarize some of the evidence implicating genetic factors in the etiology of early onset CAD as well as some of the evidence showing that genes are of importance for the population variation in several well established risk factors or protective factors for CAD. Examples of the above mechanisms underlying genetically influenced CAD risk will be given and the "variability gene concept" will be presented. Particular emphasis will be on the risk caused by a genetically determined high level of Lp(a) lipoprotein and other proven or potential genetic risk factors will be discussed. Finally, practical use of existing and forthcoming genetic information in the attempts to prevent or delay CAD will be discussed.

CORONARY ARTERY DISEASE IN FAMILIES

Several authors have reported an aggregation of CAD cases in families. Yater et al. (1948) studied CAD in men 18–39 years old and found a greater familial tendency toward heart disease among the relatives of the patients than in a control group of families. They concluded that heredity could be important for the development of CAD in young and middle-aged men. Rose (1964) found a nearly 3-fold greater mortality rate from CAD among parents of patients with myocardial infarction than among matched controls. Heyden et al. (1969) observed increased mortality from vascular diseases in parents of patients with atherosclerosis of the carotid arteries. In the Western Collaborative Group Study, incidence of CAD was associated with a history of parental CAD (Rosenman et al., 1975).

Slack and Evans (1966) studied first-degree relatives of people with CAD and controls. When death in men under age 55 and in women under age 65 was considered, the relatives of female patients with onset before age 65 showed a nearly 7-fold increase compared with the general population. Male relatives of male patients who had had CAD onset before age 55 showed an increased risk of death that was 5 times greater than in the general population. Familial clustering of CAD was especially striking for female patients. The sex differences observed were particularly suggestive of an effect of genes.

It was observed in the Tecumseh Study (Epstein, 1976) that familial aggregation of risk factors could not be successfully used to predict coronary events. This suggested that familial aggregation of disease was not exclusively mediated through familial resemblance in serum cholesterol or other risk factors analyzed. Thus, yet undiscovered familial/genetic factors seemed to account for familial aggregation of CAD cases.

Important family studies of CAD were conducted in Finland by Rissanen and Nikkilä (1977, 1979) and Rissanen (1979a,b). In the high-incidence area of North Karelia, 104 of 296 brothers of index cases had CAD as opposed to 8 of 81 brothers of control persons. CAD was observed in 36 of 294 sisters of index patients and in 6 of 96 sisters of control individuals. Cummulative risk of developing fatal or nonfatal CAD by age 65 was 4.5–fold for case brothers and 2.6–fold for cases sisters, when compared with reference sibs. The risk was highest to sibs who also had a parental history of premature CAD. Heritability estimates conducted by the Finnish workers were compatible with almost total determination of the disease by additive polygenic factors in the youngest age group (myocardial infarction prior to age 46). Also, the relatives of the youngest patients had a similar incidence of CAD in South Finland as in the high-incidence area of East Finland. This suggests that genetic determination of the disease in young people was strong enough to obliterate any regional differences in environmental/nutritional risk factors. In some of the Finnish families, the number of affected people was high enough to suggest the effect of a dominant gene that directly causes CAD.

In a study of 207 patients who had had myocardial infarction prior to age 55, and 621 controls, it was found that the highest risk ratios were associated with a positive family history of CAD (Nora et al., 1980). The highest risk was when CAD had occurred in a first-degree relative before age 55, and the second highest risk was when CAD had occurred in a first-degree relative before age 65. Importantly, CAD in a second-degree relative also increased the risk. Heritability for early onset CAD was calculated to be 0.63 when all patients and their families were considered. After elimination of 31 families in which the proband had a monogenic type of hyperlipidemia, the heritability estimate remained as high as 0.56. The risk due to a family history of early CAD was higher than that for the people in the top quintile of cholesterol levels. This finding again suggested that there were important genetic effects that were not mediated through familial resemblance in cholesterol level.

Supporting evidence emerged from the Framingham Heart Study (Snowden et al., 1982). Studying pairs of brothers, it was found that the incidence of myocardial infarction in the older brother significantly related to myocardial infarction experience in the younger brother, even after the effect of total cholesterol, systolic blood pressure and cigarette smoking had been controlled for. Again, the findings suggested that a family history of disease is an important independent predictor of myocardial infarction that is not reflected in the measured levels of total cholesterol, systolic blood pressure, or cigarette smoking. Further support that a family history of myocardial infarction is an independent risk factor for CAD was published by Friedlander et al. (1982). Finally Williams (1984) found that approximately 50% of cases of early CAD in Utah were associated with a strong familial tendency to contract this disease which was present in only 5–7% of the general population. The most recent studies of familial aggregation of early CAD usually include studies of specific genetic markers and will be commented on in connection with such markers (see below).

A series of twin studies of CAD has been reported, and a higher concordance rate in monozygotic (MZ) than in dizygotic (DZ) twin pairs has been repeatedly observed (for review, see Berg, 1983). There is evidence that genetic factors also influence the degree of CAD. In a Norwegian study of CAD patients, we found differences between high, intermediate, and low degree of familial clustering of CAD with respect to total score at coronary angiography (theoretical maximum: 50), number of coronary arteries affected (theoretical maximum: 4), and highest single score (theoretical maximum: 5). The difference between the high and low category with respect to total score was highly significant (Table 1-1).

These and other studies make it extremely difficult to escape the conclusion that there is a significant effect of genes in the etiology of CAD, at least when the disease manifests itself prior to ages 55–60 in males or ages 60–65 in females. Furthermore, the above studies clearly show that far from all of the risk resulting from having a close relative with early CAD is reflected in traditional risk factor determination. This makes it an important task to try to identify the individual genes that contribute to this risk.

FAMILIAL HYPERLIPIDEMIAS

Monogenic Hypercholesterolemia

Hypercholesterolemia with xanthomatosis is the most thoroughly examined and best understood monogenic hyperlipidemia (Müller, 1939, Fredrickson et al., 1967; Heiberg and Berg, 1976; Goldstein et al., 1972; Heiberg, 1975; Motulsky, 1976). A high serum level of low density lipoprotein (LDL) is the prominent lipoprotein abnormality in this disorder, but this lipoprotein disturbance is also found in many sporadic cases of atherosclerotic disease and also secondary to other disorders.

Table 1-1 Norwegian CAD patients: sum of scores from 10 regions of coronary arteries (total score), number of coronary arteries affected, and highest single score, from coronary angiography, according to familial occurrence of CAD*

Degree of familial clustering	N	Total score (mean)	Number of affected arteries (mean)	Highest single score (mean)
High	49	17.0[a]	2.9	4.2
Intermediate	47	15.4[b]	2.8	4.1
Low	22	10.6	2.0	2.8

* Adapted from Berg (1983).

[a] Significance of difference from low group: $p < 0.007$.

[b] Significance of difference from low group: $p < 0.05$.

Thanks to the pioneering work by Brown and Goldstein (Goldstein and Brown, 1973; Brown and Goldstein, 1974, 1976; Brown and Goldstein, 1986), it is now known in great detail what the defect is on the molecular level in autosomal dominant hypercholesterolemia. Homozygotes for familial hypercholesterolemia either completely lack functional low density lipoprotein receptors (LDLR) or have this receptor in a markedly reduced quantity so that their cells bind only up to 10% of the number of LDL molecules bound by normal genes. Heterozygotes have LDLR functional characteristics intermediate between normal homozygotes and homozygotes for familial hypercholesterolemia. The studies by Brown, Goldstein, and others have demonstrated that there is a high number of mutations at the LDLR locus that may cause monogenic hypercholesterolemia (Brown and Goldstein, 1987).

In an extensive study of familial hypercholesterolemia in a Norwegian population (Heiberg, 1975; Heiberg and Berg, 1976), a frequency of 2–3 : 1,000 was found. This frequency is in good agreement with that estimated by American workers in Seattle (Motulsky, 1976). The latter workers found that autosomal dominant hypercholesterolemia accounted for approximately 5% of the cases of myocardial infarction occurring prior to age 60. Family studies in our laboratory (Berg and Heiberg, 1976, 1977) and in two other centers (Ott et al., 1974; Elston et al., 1976) uncovered genetic linkage between the disease and a normal genetic polymorphism in the third component of complement (C3). This coassigned the LDLR locus to chromosome 19 when Whitehead et al. (1982) were able to assign the C3 locus to that chromosome (Berg et al., 1984). The LDLR locus is on the short arm of chromosome 19 (19p13.2-p13.1).

Early work in our group (Maartmann-Moe et al., 1981a) showed a significant variation (and also overlap) in LDLR function parameters in healthy people as well as in patients with autosomal dominant hypercholesterolemia. Clearly, not everybody with a defect in the LDLR function becomes equally affected. Recently, Hobbs et al. (1989) reported strong evidence that there is a dominant gene that suppresses hypercholesterolemia in occasional families with defective LDLRs. This gene is linked neither to the LDLR locus nor to the loci for apolipoprotein B (apoB) or apoE. The authors suggest that this putative gene may explain the occasional observation of normal LDL cholesterol concentrations in heterozygotes for LDL receptor mutations (Hobbs et al., 1989).

"Combined" or "Multiple Type" Hyperlipidemia

Studies in Seattle on premature CAD (Goldstein et al., 1972) led to results suggesting that as many as 20% of those who suffer a myocardial infarction prior to age 60 have a monogenic lipoprotein disorder segregating in their families. The most frequent of these disorders was a previously undetected type of hyperlipidemia which led to increased serum levels of cholesterol or triglycerides or both lipids. Motulsky (1976) has estimated the frequency of the "combined" or "multiple type" hyperlipoproteinemia to be about 1.5% in the general population. According to the Seattle workers, this hyperlipidemia occurs at least twice as frequently in survivors of myocardial infarction below age 60, as does classical familial hypercholesterolemia.

Studies in Finland (Aro, 1973; Nikkilä and Aro, 1973) of survivors of acute myocardial infarction occurring before age 50 revealed a high percentage of a similar "multiple type" hyperlipoproteinemia in patients and their family members. Confirmation of familial occurrence of "combined" hyperlipoproteinemia was also reported by Glueck et al. (1973). In their study, about half of the siblings of patients had hyperlipoproteinemia in accordance with the distribution expected for autosomal dominant inheritance. However, when the offspring of people with combined hyperlipoproteinemia were examined, a much lower proportion of affected persons was found. It has been hypothesized that the ratio of affected to unaffected persons may approach the distribution expected in autosomal dominant inheritance when the offspring of probands reach a higher age. Penetrance appears to be incomplete until the late twenties. The molecular defect in this disorder is unknown.

Familial Hypertriglyceridemia

About 5% of middle-aged survivors of myocardial infarction in Seattle appeared to have monogenic hypertriglyceridemia (Goldstein et al., 1972). The frequency of this disorder in a middle-aged population has been estimated to be about 1% (Motulsky, 1976). The relevance of this condition to CAD is not clear since in some families hypertriglyceridemia does not seem to carry an increased risk of CAD and it seems likely that the disease is heterogeneous.

As in "combined" or "multiple type" hyperlipoproteinemia, penetrance appears to be incomplete until the late twenties (Goldstein et al., 1972; Motulsky, 1976). The defect at the molecular level in the "garden variety" of familial hypertriglyceridemia is not known.

Polygenic Hypercholesterolemia

Motulsky (1976) uses this term for cases of familial clustering of hypercholesterolemia that do not follow a mendelian segregation pattern. Contrary to the situation in dominantly inherited hypercholesterolemia, the distribution of cholesterol levels in first-degree relatives of patients is unimodal. It is, however, shifted upward from the population mean toward a higher mean value.

Familial Dyslipidemic Hypertension

Williams et al. (1988) found that a disorder characterized by hypertension and dyslipidemia occurred in approximately 30% of patients with essential hypertension and appeared to follow autosomal dominant inheritance. The lipid abnormality in these families resembled familial "combined" hyperlipidemia, but in addition there seemed to be a low level of HDL. This apparently monogenic syndrome appeared to be present in 1–2% of adults in the Utah population and in 48–63% of persons who have hypertension diagnosed before age 60 when at least one of the siblings has hypertension before age 60.

If confirmed, this study shows the necessity to conduct lipid determinations in people with premature hypertension and to scrutinize blood pressure in people with early hyperlipidemias. It is to be hoped that the prognosis of these patients will be improved when care is taken to treat both their lipid abnormalities and their hypertension.

Concluding Remarks

From the information summarized above, monogenic hyperlipidemias appear to account for about 20% of the myocardial infarctions prior to age 60, but this figure may have to be adjusted upwards if the recent report concerning familial dyslipidemic hypertension is confirmed. An even greater adjustment would be needed if "genetic dyslipidemias" in a broader sense are considered. Genest et al. (1989) examined 101 probands with angiographically documented CAD prior to age 60 and their relatives. In two-thirds of the probands, a genetic dyslipidemia was identified. The dominating entities were: high level of Lp(a) lipoprotein (31.0%), combined hyperlipidemia (12.5%), and familial hypertriglyceridemia with hypo-alpha-lipoproteinemia (14.5%).

In cases of autosomal dominant disorders, the importance of providing proper counseling about the 50% risk to offspring of affected people is obvious. Dietary manipulation, or if this fails, drug treatment, should be actively offered to persons with an autosomal dominant trait rendering them susceptible to CAD (concerning Lp(a) lipoprotein, see below). The situation is much better then before for a serious condition such as monogenic hypercholesterolemia because of the excellent effect of drugs inhibiting 3-hydroxy-3-methyl-coenzyme A reductase, the rate limiting enzyme in cholesterol biosynthesis, but it is also important to fully utilize any effect achievable by dietary manipulation. Interestingly, there is evidence (e.g., from the Utah study) that people with a significant predisposition to CAD contracted the disease at an older age two or three generations ago (Williams, 1984). This suggests that dietary and lifestyle manipulation today may cause significant risk reduction or at least a significant postponement of disease development. Thus, a defeatist attitude is not justified, even in monogenic hyperlipidemias.

Although the importance of monogenic hyperlipidemias in early onset CAD is significant, most cases of myocardial infarction occurring prior to ages 55–65 do not have a monogenic hyperlipidemia or a disorder that can safely be scored as polygenic hypercholesterolemia. In the rest of this chapter, emphasis will be on CAD occurring in people without classical, inherited hyperlipidemia.

GENETIC INFLUENCE ON RISK FACTOR LEVELS

It is well known that genes affect the level of serum cholesterol in several animal species including beef cattle, squirrel monkeys, mice, and rats (for review, see Berg, 1979; Berg, 1983).

In man, the genetic influence on normal lipid levels has been studied by analysis of correlations between relatives. In Greece, Mayo et al. (1969) found significant parent-offspring and sib-sib correlations from serum cholesterol. There was no significant correlation between spouses. Their findings have been confirmed by several other workers (for review, see Berg, 1989a). Genes have also been shown to be of importance for the levels of fasting triglycerides, apolipoprotein A-I (apoA-I), apolipoprotein A-II (apoA-II), and apolipoprotein (apoB). The level of Lp(a) lipoprotein (Berg, 1963) is almost exclusively determined by genes (see below).

Several studies have indicated that genes may be of importance in the etiology of hypertension (for review, see Williams et al., 1984). We have observed high heritability for systolic as well as diastolic blood pressure (0.64 and 0.51, respectively) (Berg, 1989a). There are strong genetic determinants in obesity (Stunkard et al., 1986) and we have arrived at a surprisingly high heritability estimate for body mass index (Berg, 1989a). Examples of heritability estimates from our own laboratory are given in Table 1-2, which shows the result of studying two different series of Norwegian twins. The first series (study 1) consisted of 98 MZ and 100 same-sex DZ pairs. In this study, both traditional heritability (h^2) calculations and model fitting were carried out with essentially the same results. The second series (study 2) consisted of 156 MZ twin pairs and the within-pair correlation coefficient was, in this study, used as a heritability estimate. Although it can be argued that the within-pair correlation coefficient in MZ pairs will

Table 1-2 Estimates of heritability (h^2) of risk factors or protective factors for CAD as well as body mass index and pulse rate, from one series of Norwegian twins consisting of 98 MZ and 100 same-sex DZ pairs (study 1) and from a second series of 156 MZ twin pairs (study 2)

	Heritability (h^2) estimate	
Parameter	Study 1	Study 2
Total cholesterol	0.34	0.68
Fasting triglycerides	0.40	0.46
ApoB	0.66	0.64
ApoA-I	0.53	0.55
ApoA-II	0.69	0.68
Lp(a) lipoprotein	1.0	~1.0
Systolic blood pressure	—	0.64
Diastolic blood pressure	—	0.51
Body mass index	—	0.76
Pulse rate	—	0.59

overestimate heritability, the results are remarkably similar between the two series with respect to heritability of apolipoprotein levels. Heritability estimates for lipid and apoproteins from the two studies are shown in Table 1-2, together with heritability estimates for blood pressure, body mass index and pulse rate, from study 2. The genes contributing to level of risk factors or protective factors, however, are generally unknown (see below).

RANDOM GENETIC MARKERS, LIPID LEVELS, AND ATHEROSCLEROSIS

Studies of random markers uncovered association with lipid levels more than 20 years ago (Mayo et al., 1969, 1971), and in an extensive analysis Sing and Orr (1976) confirmed and extended the early studies of random marker associations (associations between cholesterol and the ABO and Secretor blood group systems, and the Hp and Gm serum type systems were firmly established). Of the associations discovered in the latter study, the association between lipid level and the haptoglobin serum type system appears to be between HDL cholesterol and haptoglobin variants, rather than between haptoglobin and atherogenic LDL cholesterol (Børresen et al., 1987). The locus for the enzume lecithin : cholesterol acyl transferase (LCAT) is very closely linked to haptoglobin (on chromosome 16) and it seems plausible that the association between HDL cholesterol level and haptoglobin was in fact caused by variation at the LCAT locus or at the locus for some other component important in lipid metabolism that is closely linked to the haptoglobin locus.

Although associations between risk factor levels or overt disease, and random genetic markers confirmed that genetic factors are of importance in atherosclerosis, the studies with random genetic markers offered little hope of a deeper understanding of the mechanisms underlying atherosclerotic disorders. The rationale behind the study of genetic markers with no known relationship to lipid metabolism or disease mechanisms was the hope that they could uncover effects of closely linked loci whose products were involved in atherogenesis or thrombogenesis.

THE CANDIDATE GENE APPROACH

Much more interesting than the study of random markers, is the candidate gene approach. With respect to atherosclerosis and CAD, a candidate gene is any gene whose protein product is:

   involved in lipoprotein structure, lipoprotein metabolism or lipid metabolism;
   involved in thrombogenesis, thrombolysis or fibrinolysis;
   involved in regulation of blood flow in coronary arteries;
   involved in regulation of blood pressure;
   involved in reverse cholesterol transport;

present in atherosclerotic lesions;
involved in the regulation of growth of atherosclerotic lesions;
involved in the early development of coronary arteries.

The first time the candidate gene approach was applied (although the term candidate gene had not yet been introduced) was in the early 1970s when direct association between genetically determined Lp(a) lipoprotein (Berg, 1963) and premature CAD was discovered (Berg et al., 1974).

In the mid 1970s, association between lipid levels and allotypic Ag variants of LDL were uncovered (Berg et al., 1976) and in the late 1970s it was demonstrated that the apoE polymorphism is associated with cholesterol levels in the general population (Utermann et al., 1979). Thus, the candidate gene approach applied at the apolipoprotein level led to the discovery of lipid as well as disease associations.

The availability of DNA technology has greatly increased the possibilities for identifying single genes that contribute to the heritability of risk factor levels and to genetic predisposition to CAD. In this connection, attention has until recently been focused on apolipoprotein genes in which many restriction fragment length polymorphisms (RFLPs) have been uncovered. Recently, there has been an increased interest in also studying DNA variation at loci for lipases and for components involved in "reverse cholesterol transport" (see below).

THE VARIABILITY GENE CONCEPT

Marker genes exhibiting association with absolute risk factor levels may for convenience be referred to as level genes. We have postulated that genes may be of importance for lipids and other CAD risk factors not only by contributing to absolute risk factor levels, but also by determining the framework within which nutritional and other environmental factors may cause risk factor variation. Such genes may be referred to as variability genes to distinguish them from level genes.

We have developed a method to detect variability gene effects based on the study of MZ twins (Berg, 1981, 1984; Magnus et al., 1981a). Since MZ twins have identical genes, any difference between the two members of a pair in a quantitative biological parameter must be caused by environmental, lifestyle, or nutritional factors. A gene affecting variability should therefore be detectable by comparing the mean within-pair difference in a quantitative parameter between MZ pairs who have and MZ pairs who lack the gene under study. If a variability gene has a permissive effect, greater within-pair difference would be observed in MZ pairs possessing than in those lacking the gene, whereas the opposite would be true for a variability gene with a restrictive effect. This method may at present be the best available approach to gene-environment interactions.

Using random genetic markers, we documented several years ago that it is realistic to search for variability genes, and that at least some of them have no level gene effect (Berg, 1981, 1984; Magnus et al., 1981a). We found significant results, more frequently than expected by chance alone, and it was likely that one or more of the results reflected true biological phenomena (Berg, 1984). We found evidence for a restrictive effect of the M allele in the MNSs blood group system (or genes at a closely linked locus), and of the Jk^b gene in the Kidd blood group system, on cholesterol variability. Neither of the blood group systems had any effect on absolute lipid levels. In an independent, new series we recently confirmed the effect of Kidd blood group genes (or closely linked genes) on cholesterol variability (Berg, 1988). At present, we are searching for variability gene effects at several candidate loci, using DNA technology (see below).

RELEVANCE OF THE VARIABILITY GENE CONCEPT TO HEALTH AND DISEASE IN MAN

An early study of cholesterol variability in individual persons over a 5-year period showed that everybody who developed CAD had a high degree of variability, suggesting that the amount of variation observed in risk factors may be clinically relevant (Groover et al., 1960).

It has been known for almost 20 years that strain differences in blood lipid response to dietary cholesterol intake exist in animal species (for review, see Berg, 1979). Terms such as hyperresponder and hyporesponder have been introduced to describe phenotypes. These strain differences are almost certainly genetically determined. Differences in response between humans to dietary cholesterol have also been reported, but until recently the issue was less clear for man than for various animal species. However, Katan and his coworkers have recently demonstrated that hyporesponders and hyperresponders to dietary cholesterol exist in man and that these traits persist, over many years at least (Beynen and Katan, 1985; Katan et al., 1986; Katan and Beynen, 1987). They calculated that if the mean cholesterol response to a certain dietary cholesterol load is 0.58 mmol/l, then the 16% of subjects who are least susceptible to diet will experience a cholesterol response of only 0.29 mmol/l or less, whereas the 16% of subjects who are most susceptible to diet will have a response of 0.87 mmol/l or more. Thus, important individual differences with respect to response to dietary cholesterol are probably present in man and it is plausible that hyporesponders and hyperresponders exist in the same way as they do in animals. The existence of significant differences between individuals in response to fat intake makes it necessary to apply more dynamic genetic approaches to CAD risk studies than traditional analysis of marker gene associations with absolute lipid or apolipoprotein levels. Variability gene analyses should be included in such approaches.

A person's status with respect to being a hyporesponder or hyperresponder may well by as relevant to his or her risk to develop atherosclerosis as are absolute risk factor levels. Therefore, it is important to try to identify variability genes—genes that contribute to the hyporesponder or hyperresponder trait.

It is likely that gene-environment interactions are of importance for a wide variety of common disorders. With respect to CAD risk, it appears likely that a person's total genetic risk depends on his or her *combination* of level genes and variability genes (Table 1-3).

Lp(a) LIPOPROTEIN AND CAD

Introduction

The Lp(a) lipoprotein is a distinct class of serum lipoproteins identified by immunological methods in 1963 (Berg, 1963). Following certain absorption procedures, individual sera could be scored as Lp(a+) or Lp(a−) in agar gel double immunodiffusion experiments, and Lp phenotype was shown to be genetically determined (Berg, 1963, 1968; Berg and Mohr, 1963). The Lp(a) lipoprotein was detected also in the sera of nonhuman primates and behaved as a genetic trait also in those species (Berg, 1969).

Several workers performing electrophoretic analysis of serum lipo-proteins encountered "atypical" lipoproteins in the late 1960s and early 1970s. The "sinking pre-β-lipoprotein" of Rider and coworkers exhibited autosomal dominant inheritance and was shown to be identical to the Lp(a) lipoprotein (Rider et al., 1970; Heiberg and Berg, 1974). The same was the case for the "pre-β_1 lipoprotein" of Dahlén (1974). Rittner (1971) prepared concentrated fractions of lipoprotein of density 1.063–1.10 and found genetic variants using disc electrophoresis. A strong, although not abso-lute association with immunologically detected Lp(a) lipoprotein was un-covered. It is unknown if the variation studied by Rittner is related to the isoforms of the polypeptide chain carrying the Lp(a) antigen (see below) reported recently by Utermann and his coworkers (Utermann et al., 1987; 1988a, 1988b).

It was clear at a very early stage that differences in Lp(a) lipoprotein quantity existed between sera of phenotype Lp(a+) (Berg, 1964, 1971). In the late 1960s, several workers detected small quantities of Lp(a) lipo-

Table 1-3 Proposed, genetically determined, CAD risk resulting from the combina-tion of genes affecting level and variability, respectively, of CAD risk factors*

Risk factor level specified by level genes	Total genetic risk when variability genes are	
	Permissive	Restrictive
High	High, but reducible	Very high
Average	Average, but changeable	Average
Low	Low, but changeable	Very low

* Adapted from Berg (1987b).

protein also in serum of people who typed as Lp(a−) in the traditional double immunodiffusion analyses.

Quantitative Studies of Lp(a) Lipoprotein

The existence of sera that produced only very weak precipitin bands in double immunodiffusion experiments, together with the finding of small amounts of Lp(a) lipoprotein in sera which scored as Lp(a−) in the traditional test system, made it necessary to conduct quantitative experiments with Lp(a) lipoprotein. In particular, it became important to examine the relationship between phenotype by double immunodiffusion experiments and quantity of Lp(a) lipoprotein. Studies by Schultz et al. (1974) and by Sing et al. (1974), using a sensitive radioimmunoassay, uncovered a clear relationship between traditional Lp(a) phenotyping and Lp(a) lipoprotein level. We have based our own quantitative Lp(a) lipoprotein studies on quantitative immunoelectrophoresis with high quality antisera incorporated into an agarose gel. The reference serum is standardized against pure Lp(a) lipoprotein fractions whose protein content has been determined by the micro-Kjeldahl method.

The relationship between scoring of Lp(a) phenotype by double immunodiffusion and quantitative determination with polyvalent antiserum is illustrated in Table 1-4, which shows the result of a blindly conducted study (Berg, 1990a). All serum samples belonging to the top quartile of Lp(a) lipoprotein concentrations were detected as normal positive reactions in double immunodiffusion. Some 5% of the persons in the 51–75th percentile were also detected, but no sample belonging to the two lower quartiles was present among the normal positive reactions. Mean Lp(a) lipoprotein levels were significantly higher in all categories of positive

Table 1-4 Distribution of 160 unrelated individuals with respect to Lp(a) lipoprotein phenotype determined by agarose gel double immunodiffusion technique and quartile of Lp(a) lipoprotein concentration*

Lp(a) phenotype	Lp(a) lipoprotein percentile			Total number
	0–25	26–75	76–100	
Lp(a−)	39	70	0	109
Lp(a + w)	1	8	0	9
Lp(a+)	0	2	10	12
Lp(a++)	0	0	30	30
Total	40	80	40	160

* Adapted from Berg (1990a).
$\chi^2 = 160.2$, 9 d.f., $p < 0.0001$.
Lp(a−) = no precipitin band.
Lp(a + w) = weak or doubtful precipitin band.
Lp(a+), Lp(a++) = definite precipitin bands, but with strength difference.

reactions than in people who typed as Lp(a−) in double immunodiffusion experiments (Table 1-5). This recent study again confirms excellent agreement between phenotyping by double immunodiffusion and quantitative Lp(a) lipoprotein determination and shows that normal positive reactions identify the samples with the highest Lp(a) lipoprotein levels.

Lp(a) Lipoprotein as a Quantitative Genetic Trait

The quantitative analyses conducted in the early 1970s by Schultz et al. (1974) and Sing et al. (1974) provided strong evidence for single locus control of Lp(a) lipoprotein concentration. In the Honolulu Heart Study, quantitative Lp(a) lipoprotein determinations were blindly conducted in two different laboratories. The agreement between results for the two laboratories was extremely good and this large study provided strong confirmation of single locus control of Lp(a) lipoprotein concentrations (Morton et al., 1985). Several twin studies have been conducted and all have resulted in heritability estimates of unity or very close to unity.

The total body of evidence leads to the conclusion that Lp(a) lipoprotein concentration, measured in healthy individuals with adequate test systems, is almost exclusively genetically determined by major genes at a single locus. The close relationship between Lp(a) lipoprotein phenotyping by double immunodiffusion technique and quantitative determination of Lp(a) lipoprotein level appears to explain the early findings by agar or agarose gel double immunodiffusion of autosomal dominant inheritance of the Lp(a+) phenotype, with very few exceptions.

Table 1-5   Lp(a) lipoprotein levels determined by quantitative immunoelectrophoresis in 160 unrelated Norwegians belonging to 4 scoring categories for Lp(a) lipoprotein phenotype by agarose gel double immunodiffusion technique. The protein content of the pre Lp(a) lipoprotein solution used for standardization had been determined by the micro-Kjeldahl technique and the levels (mg/dl) are given as protein

		Lp(a) lipoprotein	
Lp(a) phenotype	No. of individuals	Mean	S.D.
Lp(a−)	109	3.3[a]	3.1
Lp(a + w)	9	6.9[b]	3.7
Lp(a+)	12	15.7[c]	4.1
Lp(a++)	30	26.9[c]	7.3

[a] p = 0.001 for difference from Lp(a + w) group, p < 0.0001 for differences from other groups.
[b] p = 0.001 for difference from Lp(a−) group, p < 0.0001 for differences from other groups.
[c] p < 0.0001 for differences from other groups.
Lp(a-) = no precipitin band.
Lp(a + w) = weak or doubtful precipitin band.
Lp(a+), Lp(a++) = definite precipitin band, but with strength difference.

Lp(a) Lipoprotein as a Genetic Risk Factor for CAD

Studies from the 1970s in Scandinavia (Berg et al., 1974; Dahlén et al., 1976; Frick et al., 1978; Berg, 1979) that established a clear correlation between Lp(a) lipoprotein and CAD have been confirmed in many subsequent series and a high Lp(a) lipoprotein level is firmly established as a significant, independent genetic risk factor for CAD (Berg, 1979, 1983, 1990a, 1990b; Brown and Goldstein, 1987).

This is well illustrated by the findings of Rhoads et al. (1986) of a population attributable risk of 28% for men in the top quartile of Lp(a) lipoprotein levels to contract myocardial infarction prior to age 60. These workers also found a significant effect of a high Lp(a) lipoprotein level on myocardial infarction risk in the 60–69 years age group. Durrington et al. (1988) reported that practically all familial clustering of cases of premature CAD, in the absence of monogenic hyperlipidemia, was caused by a high Lp(a) lipoprotein level. We found a high Lp(a) lipoprotein level significantly more frequently in people with CAD among their close relatives than in people whose families did not exhibit early CAD cases (Berg et al., 1979).

The reason for the association between Lp(a) lipoprotein and CAD is not known. Maartmann-Moe and Berg (1981) did not find that unlabeled Lp(a) lipoprotein competed with labeled LDL in LDL receptor function analyses of cultured fibroblasts. Furthermore, they found no significant difference in Lp(a) lipoprotein uptake between cultured fibroblasts from healthy people and heterozygotes or homozygotes for familial hypercholesterolemia (Maartmann-Moe and Berg, 1981). Finally, HMG-CoA reductase inhibitors that strongly reduce LDL levels have no effect on Lp(a) lipoprotein level. These observations, together with linkage analyses that show that a high serum level of Lp(a) lipoprotein is determined by a locus extremely closely linked to the plasminogen locus (see below) argue against a major role of the LDL receptor in the catabolism of Lp(a) lipoprotein. However, the matter is not quite resolved. In transgenic mice overexpressing the human LDLR receptor, accelerated catabolism of Lp(a) lipoprotein was observed (Hofmann et al., 1990) whereas Neven et al. (1990) studying rhesus monkeys found evidence that the LDLR receptor plays no major role in Lp(a) lipoprotein metabolism. Lp(a) lipoprotein level is independent of cholesterol concentration when total and LDL cholesterol values are corrected for cholesterol present in the Lp(a) lipoprotein particles themselves. Therefore, it is unlikely that interference with LDL receptor function explains the atherogenic properties of Lp(a) lipoprotein.

Lp(a) lipoprotein particles have been detected in atherosclerotic lesions by other workers (Walton, 1972; Rath et al., 1989) and the amount correlates with the serum concentration of Lp(a) lipoprotein. Under conditions resembling those prevailing in the arterial wall, we have shown that the Lp(a) lipoprotein particle very easily forms aggregates (Dahlén et al., 1978).

In continuation of pioneering biochemical studies of Lp(a) lipoprotein by Fless et al. (1984, 1986), workers in Chicago and San Francisco reported in 1987 that partial amino acid sequence had shown that the apolipoprotein carrying the Lp(a) antigen has extensive homology to plasminogen (Eaton et al., 1987). Later that year, the same group of workers reported cloning and complete sequence determination of cDNA representing the Lp(a) polypeptide chain (McLean et al., 1987). The homology to plasminogen was shown to be most impressive.

The extensive homology to plasminogen raised the distinct possibility that the association of Lp(a) lipoprotein to CAD is caused by interference with thrombolytic/fibrinolytic processes. In vitro studies by several groups have yielded results that agree with this notion. Thus, Harpel et al. (1989) have demonstrated affinity between Lp(a) lipoprotein and protease-modified fibrinogen or fibrin, and Hajjar et al. (1989) have reported Lp(a) lipoprotein modulation of endothelial cell surface fibrinolysis. Miles et al. (1989) observed Lp(a) lipoprotein competition for plasminogen receptors by molecular mimicry. Conclusive evidence for in vivo interference with thrombolytic/fibrinolytic processes is missing. Nevertheless, the extensive homology between the LPA and plasminogen genes seems to provide a long-sought bridge between atherogenesis and thrombogenesis (Brown and Goldstein, 1987).

Molecular Genetics of the Lp(a) Lipoprotein

Extensive biochemical studies in many laboratories have shown that the Lp(a) antigen(s) resides in a long polypeptide chain (the Lp(a) polypeptide chain or the Lp(a) apolipoprotein) which in the intact Lp(a) lipoprotein particle is bound to apoB by a disulfide bond. Utermann et al. (1987) have demonstrated that isoforms of the Lp(a) polypeptide chain exist. It seems that these isoforms may vary in size from 200,000–300,000 to 600,000–700,000 Daltons.

Table 1-6 shows a comparison between the gene for the Lp(a) polypeptide chain based on the report by McLean et al. (1987) and the plasminogen gene.

Except for the resulting size difference, the most striking difference between plasminogen and Lp(a) polypeptide chain is that the latter contains a high number of a structure homologous to kringle IV of plasminogen—37 copies in the sample reported by McLean et al. (1987). The extensive homology suggests that the gene for the Lp(a) polypeptide chain has developed from the plasminogen gene.

We have uncovered quantitative genetic variation in the Lp(a) gene, employing probes developed by the Genentech group (McLean et al., 1987). This variation is also detectable with probes that only detect DNA representing kringle IV. Under suitable conditions there is no interference from plasminogen (Kondo and Berg, 1990). The quantitative variation can be detected with several different restriction enzymes, most likely reflecting differences between individuals in number of kringle IV repeats,

Table 1-6 Comparison between Lp(a) polypeptide chain and plasminogen*

Parameter	Plasminogen	Lp(a)
Amino acids in mature protein	791	4,529
Signal peptide	1	1
"Tail" region	1	0
Kringle[a] I	1	0
Kringle II	1	0
Kringle III	1	0
Kringle IV	1	37[b]
Kringle V	1	1
"Protease" region	1	1
Cleavage site for TPA	1	0

* Based on the cDNA data of McLean et al. (1987).

[a] Cysteine-rich sequence of 80-114 amino acids.

[b] In sample analyzed.

the phenomenon likely to cause the Lp(a) apolipoprotein isoform polymorphism (Berg, 1990b; Kondo and Berg, 1990). If varying numbers of kringle IV repeats underlie the protein isoforms, DNA analysis will probably be the method of choice for detecting this genetic variation. We have also uncovered a restriction fragment length polymorphism in the Lp(a) gene, most likely residing in the 3' part of the gene or in the DNA area flanking it. This polymorphism is not detectable with a kringle IV probe, under appropriate conditions (Berg et al., 1990).

The detection of extensive homology between the LPA and plasminogen genes and the suggestion of a close evolutionary relationship (McLean et al., 1987) led several groups to conduct genetic linkage studies between Lp(a) lipoprotein and plasminogen. Weitkamp et al. (1988) analyzed families whose members had been scored with respect to Lp(a) phenotype by double immunodiffusion (as stated above, this technique primarily detects the people with the highest Lp(a) lipoprotein level), and a plasminogen polymorphism at the protein level. Although they observed cases of apparent recombination, a maximum lod score of 12.7 was obtained. It is likely that several of the apparent recombinants were the result of misclassification of either a child or a parent by the double immunodiffusion technique, as suggested by the authors themselves. The close linkage reported by Weitkamp et al. (1988) to a definite single-gene polymorphism, forms definite evidence that the majority of the variation observed when the original test method is used is caused by genes at one single locus. The detected linkage shows that data based on double immunodiffusion alone carry important genetic information on this single-locus trait.

Drayna et al. (1988) analyzed an extensive Utah kindred where high levels of Lp(a) lipoprotein segregated with respect to Lp(a) lipoprotein isoforms and a DNA polymorphism at the plasminogen locus. The peak lod score between the isoforms and DNA polymorphism at the plasminogen locus was 3.8 at recombination fraction zero. The strength of the linkage between plasminogen and Lp(a) would have been the same if Lp(a) lipoprotein levels had been used instead of isoforms.

We studied linkage between Lp(a) lipoprotein and a SacI RFLP at the plasminogen locus, using Lp(a) lipoprotein level to score variation at the Lp(a) locus (Berg, 1990b). We selected nuclear families where an Lp(a) lipoprotein level in the top quartile of the population distribution segregated from only one of the parents and where the occurrence of children with very low Lp(a) lipoprotein levels showed that the parent with a high Lp(a) lipoprotein level was heterozygous for a "high" gene. Lp(a) lipoprotein level segregated as an autosomal dominant trait in all families chosen in this way. Data on the families that were informative with respect to linkage between Lp(a) lipoprotein and the SacI RFLP at the plasminogen locus were submitted to lod score analysis. There was no evidence of recombination in either sex. The total lod score arising from such families is now 7.5 for recombination fraction zero (Table 1-7). This firmly establishes linkage between the plasminogen locus and the locus determining Lp(a) lipoprotein level. The true recombination fraction between the two loci may be very small, with 95% confidence limits of the recombination fraction of 0.001 and 0.0088 for the total series. Since both categories of homozygotes in the plasminogen polymorphism were observed in the top as well as in the bottom quartile of Lp(a) lipoprotein concentrations (as well as in the remaining two quartiles), Lp(a) lipoprotein level is not determined by genes at the plasminogen locus and the two loci are not so closely linked that there is absolute allelic association (Table 1-8). This shows that DNA variation at the plasminogen locus is not an adequate instrument to study genetic variation at the Lp(a) locus.

The above studies definitely establish close linkage between plasminogen, and Lp(a) lipoprotein level and Lp(a) lipoprotein phenotype as scored by double immunodiffusion technique. The linkage data strongly suggest that Lp(a) lipoprotein level and Lp(a) phenotype reflect effects of genes at one single locus (the LPA locus). These results are definite proof that the Lp(a) lipoprotein is governed by one single Mendelian locus determining Lp(a) lipoprotein level, immunologically determined phenotype, and isoforms. The locus must be on chromosome 6 in the area 6q25-6q27 where the plasminogen locus is known to be (Swisshelm et al., 1985; Murray et al., 1985, 1987).

Table 1-7 Lod scores for the Lp(a) lipoprotein–plasminogen relationship

Segregation from	Recombination fraction					
	0.00	0.05	0.10	0.20	0.30	0.40
Males	2.71	2.34	1.97	1.25	0.62	0.17
Females	4.82	4.28	3.73	2.58	1.42	0.43
Total	7.53	6.62	5.70	3.83	2.04	0.60

Table 1-8 Distribution of 143 unrelated individuals with respect to quartile of sex and age adjusted Lp(a) lipoprotein concentration and genotype in a DNA polymorphism at the plasminogen locus detectable with the restriction enzyme SacI*

Plasminogen genotype	Lp(a) lipoprotein percentile				Total number
	0–25	26–50	51–75	76–100	
1–1	6	3	4	2	15
1–2	21	22	13	11	67
2–2	9	11	18	23	61
Total	36	36	35	36	143

* Adapted from Berg (1989a).
$\chi^2 = 15.96$, 6 d.f., p = 0.01.

Concerning Methods for Lp(a) Lipoprotein Measurements

Currently, the method of choice for Lp(a) lipoprotein determination for identifying people with increased CAD risk is quantitative immunoelectrophoresis with polyvalent antiserum of high quality (Fig. 1-1). However, traditional, standardized double immunodiffusion technique will identify people with the highest Lp(a) lipoprotein levels, particularly those in the top quartile of the population distribution. Accordingly, those at high CAD risk are identified also in the original phenotyping system. With absorbed, high quality antiserum the problem of cross reactivity with plasminogen, apoB, LDL or any other serum component can be eliminated. In quantitative immunoelectrophoresis, the observer actually sees the product of the antigen/antibody reaction as the precipitin "rocket." The single rocket we observe in our standardized test system shows that the Lp(a) lipoprotein determination is not disturbed by crossreaction with other components.

Many workers consider quantitative immunoelectrophoresis too laborious to be used in a population screening or in a routine clinical laboratory dependent on automation. However, with the solid evidence that a high Lp(a) lipoprotein level is a significant risk factor for CAD, it is most desirable that quantitative Lp(a) lipoprotein determination becomes much more widely used. It is therefore understandable that several research or commercial groups are working hard at developing alternative ways to determine Lp(a) lipoprotein levels. There is every reason to hope that such efforts will be successful in the future. Problems with crossreactivity with plasminogens will have to be solved. If monoclonal antibodies are used, one would have to be certain that the reagent detects all Lp(a) isoforms equally well. Purified Lp(a) lipoprotein of serum that has one particular isoform or combination of isoforms may not be valid as a reference solution to determine Lp(a) lipoprotein level in samples from people with other isoforms.

Because of the above problems we remain skeptical of any new test system or new batches of antiserum and other reagents that have not been

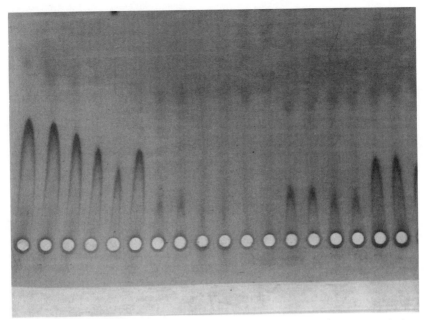

Figure 1-1 Quantitative immunoelectrophoresis to determine the amount of atherogenic Lp(a) lipoprotein. Serum from individual persons were introduced into the circular wells in an agarose gel containing highly specific antiserum to Lp(a) lipoprotein, and submitted to electrophoresis. The distance that Lp(a) lipoprotein can travel in the agarose depends on its concentration. The area under the precipitin "rocket" reflects the serum concentration of Lp(a) lipoprotein. Large differences between human sera in Lp(a) lipoprotein concentration can be observed.

clearly demonstrated to give the same results as studies with high quality antiserum in quantitative immunoelectrophoresis.

The problem of valid quantitative determination of Lp(a) lipoprotein by means of enzyme-linked immunosorbent assay (ELISA) or other techniques that are not based on an observable precipitin reaction has been the subject of much discussion. In one such discussion, it became clear that one of the commercially available kits for easy Lp(a) lipoprotein quantification also detects plasminogen. The need for careful quality control can hardly be overemphasized.

Can Risk Caused by High Lp(a) Lipoprotein Level be Modified?

The level of Lp(a) lipoprotein remains remarkably constant, at least over a great many years, and probably throughout life. It is not changed by dietary manipulation of LDL level, and with the exception of niacin (Gurakar et al., 1985), none of the lipid reducing drugs change Lp(a) lipoprotein levels. The absence of any effect of 3-hydroxy-3-methylglutaryl coenzyme A (HMGCoA) reductase inhibitors is particularly noteworthy since it confirms that Lp(a) lipoprotein and LDL are metabolically independent. There has been one report (Jürgens et al., 1989) of significant *increase* in Lp(a) lipoprotein level during HMGCoA reductase inhibitor treatment. This report is at variance with other information. In our own studies we found no effect of even the highest doses of HMGCoA reductase inhibitor on Lp(a) lipoprotein level (Berg and Leren, 1989). Thus, if HMGCoA reductase inhibitors can increase Lp(a) lipoprotein level, this must be a rare occurrence that should not cause physicians to withhold such treatment if otherwise needed. As an extra precaution, Lp(a) lipoprotein measurements may be conducted before and two or three times during treatment with HMGCoA reductase inhibitors.

Armstrong and coworkers (1986) have reported that increased LDL concentration markedly increases the risk of CAD due to elevated Lp(a) lipoprotein level. Although Lp(a) lipoprotein is not associated with total or LDL cholesterol following correction for cholesterol in the Lp(a) lipoprotein particle itself, it is not surprising that the CAD risk conferred by a high Lp(a) lipoprotein level is even higher in the presence of a high level of total or LDL cholesterol. It is tempting to speculate that the combined high risk may be caused by an unfavorable LDL level contributing to atherogenesis (together with Lp(a) lipoprotein) and a high level of Lp(a) lipoprotein affecting processes related to fibrinolysis/thrombolysis in arteries becoming atherosclerotic. If high Lp(a) lipoprotein levels are better tolerated when LDL is low, the logical conclusion would be to lower LDL cholesterol as much as possible by diet or drugs in people with a high level of Lp(a) lipoprotein. The HMGCoA reductase inhibitors would be the best candidates for drug treatment to lower LDL cholesterol in people with a high Lp(a) lipoprotein level.

The significant fall in CAD frequency in several European countries during World War II was so pronounced that it is also likely that people with a strong genetic predisposition to CAD, including most of those with a high Lp(a) lipoprotein level, escaped disease during that period. This provides hope that changes in those risk factors that can be manipulated will have a protective effect even in people with a high level of Lp(a) lipoprotein.

Practical Application of Existing Knowledge on Lp(a) Lipoprotein

Lp(a) lipoprotein level can already be measured in childhood and mass screening in early adult life is possible. The purpose of such screening would be to make it possible for people who want the screening and who want to assume responsibility for their own health, to institute as efficient preventive measures as possible, if the screening were to uncover increased CAD risk.

In clinical situations, Lp(a) lipoprotein should be determined in all cases of premature CAD (prior to 55–60 years of age in men or 60–65 in women). If a high Lp(a) lipoprotein level is detected, determination of Lp(a) lipoprotein concentration should be made in first-degree relatives of the patient, and the family should be alerted to the possibility that more distant relatives might also benefit from Lp(a) lipoprotein determination. Active preventative efforts should be instituted in every person who is found to have a high Lp(a) lipoprotein level (see below).

NORMAL GENETIC VARIATION AT CANDIDATE LOCI, RISK FACTORS, AND CORONARY ARTERY DISEASE

As mentioned above, study of normal genetic variation at the lipoprotein level has uncovered association between normal genes at candidate loci and lipid levels (the allotypic Ag variation in LDL and the apoE polymorphism) as well as overt CAD (the Lp(a) lipoprotein polymorphism). The developments with respect to DNA technology have greatly improved the potential to study genetic variation at candidate loci. Numerous candidate genes such as the apolipoprotein genes have been cloned and RFLPs at their loci detected. Several studies trying to correlate DNA variation at apolipoprotein loci to lipid levels or CAD have been published. Findings by different research groups have not always been in agreement and there are several potential sources of errors. With the numerous analyses that are being conducted, apparently positive results must occur by chance alone. Ethnic heterogeneity may cause problems and make the comparison between cases and controls invalid. Ascertainment biases may be difficult to identify. No detailed discussion will be offered of inconsistencies between studies.

The following review of published reports will be highly selective rather than comprehensive, focusing on matters that we find particularly interesting and promising.

Genes at the LDL Receptor Locus

Several years ago, our group reported a significant effect of genes on the activity of LDLR in cultured cells from healthy people (Magnus et al., 1981a,b). A limited number of normal genes at the LDL receptor locus appeared to contribute to the population distribution of LDLR activity (Maartmann-Moe et al., 1981a). An important question arising from the above findings was whether normal alleles at the LDLR locus contribute to the population variation of lipid or apolipoprotein concentrations in serum. A negative corrrelation between LDLR activity and cholesterol level suggested that such an effect may be detectable (Maartmann-Moe et al., 1981b). Using a PvuII restriction site polymorphism at the LDLR locus, we have tried to uncover effects of normal genes at this locus on lipid levels.

We found significantly higher total and LDL cholesterol levels in homozygotes for absence of the PvuII restriction site than in people possessing the restriction site (Pedersen and Berg, 1988). There was no effect on triglyceride level. We have since confirmed the effect of normal genes at the LDLR locus on total and LDL cholesterol in an independent study (Pedersen and Berg, 1990). We conclude that our suggestion, made many years ago, that normal alleles at the LDLR locus may affect lipid levels was valid. The polymorphism studied is in an intron and it could therefore not by itself reflect structural differences in the gene product. There is, however, extensive linkage disequilibrium in the LDLR gene and the association must be caused by linkage disequilibrium between the PvuII restriction site and functionally important domains.

Genetic Variation in the ApoA-I–ApoC-III–ApoA-IV Gene Cluster

The first indication that DNA variants at the apoA-I locus may be related to atherosclerosis came from studies of two patients with very low levels of high-density lipoprotein and deficiency of apoA-I and apoC-III, both of whom were shown to be homozygous for a defect in the apoA-I gene (Karathanasis et al., 1983a,b). The underlying genetic anomaly is extremely rare so this was not an example of normal genes contributing to CAD risk.

Rees and coworkers (1983, 1985, 1986) reported association between hypertriglyceridemia and an RFLP in the apoA-I–apoC-III gene cluster demonstrable with restriction enzyme SstI. Shoulders and coworkers (1986) found that this polymorphism was also associated with hypercholesterolemia in the absence of an LDLR defect. Kessling and coworkers (1985, 1986) could not confirm the association between the SstI polymorphism and hypertriglyceridemia but found indications of association between hypertriglyceridemia and a polymorphism detectable with the restriction enzyme XmnI. We have evidence suggestive of variability gene effect detectable by the XmnI polymorphism, a normal gene identified by presence of the XmnI site appearing to have permissive effect on cholesterol variability (Berg, 1989a).

A DNA polymorphism detectable with the restriction endonuclease PstI in the area flanking the human apoA-I gene at its 3' end was reported by Ordovas and coworkers (1986) to be associated with premature CAD and familial hypo-alpha-lipoproteinemia. A 3.3 kilobase (kb) fragment appeared in 3–4% of healthy people and in 32% of 88 patients who had suffered severe CAD before age 60. The report is as yet unconfirmed. If confirmed it would mean that people possessing the 3.3 kb fragment have a significantly higher risk for early CAD than people lacking that DNA fragment.

Buraczynska and her coworkers (1986) have reported an association between an apoA-I related DNA polymorphism detectable with the restriction enzyme EcoRI and CAD. The polymorphic EcoRI site was present in less than 10% of healthy controls and in 47% of people with atherosclerosis.

Ferns and coworkers (1985) reported higher frequency in postinfarction patients than in controls of a polymorphic SstI restriction site. However, the question of whether or not there is an association between the SstI polymorphism and hyperlipidemia or CAD remains unsettled (Morris and Price, 1985; Price et al., 1986; Vella et al., 1985).

Genetic Variation at the ApoB Locus

Law et al. (1986) found significantly higher triglyceride levels in people possessing a polymorphic XbaI restriction site within the apoB coding sequence than in those lacking the site. There was also a trend toward higher total cholesterol levels. Berg (1986) confirmed the association with cholesterol and triglycerides. Talmud and Humphries (1986) also found an effect of presence of the XbaI restriction site on cholesterol level. In all three studies, people who were homozygous for absence of the restriction site had lower lipid levels than homozygotes or heterozygotes for presence of the site. Several workers have confirmed the association between this DNA polymorphism and lipid levels.

Thus, there appears to be little doubt that normal genes detected at the XbaI restriction site polymorphism contribute to the population variation in total and LDL cholesterol. The XbaI polymorphism is a silent, third-base mutation corresponding to amino acid 2,488 in the mature apoB and therefore does not cause structural changes to apoB. The association must be caused by linkage disequilibrium between the XbaI site and functionally important domains. The XbaI polymorphism at the apoB locus is illustrated in Figure 1-2. Hegele et al. (1986) reported association between alleles at three RFLPs in the apoB gene with myocardial infarction. In their series, cholesterol, triglycerides, LDL cholesterol, or apoB levels did not differ significantly between patients and controls, whereas significant differences were found with respect to HDL cholesterol, apoA-I, and apoA-II levels. Thus, lower levels of HDL and its apolipoproteins appear to be a characteristic of this patient group rather than a significantly increased level of LDL lipids or apoB. Despite the association with myocardial infarction uncovered in this study, no association was detected by these authors between DNA variants at the apoB locus and lipid or apolipoprotein levels. Surprisingly, the association detected was between myocardial infarction and the variant in the XbaI polymorphism that other workers have found to be associated with *lower* levels of total and LDL cholesterol as well as triglycerides. This association between normal genes at the apoB locus and myocardial infarction has not yet been unequivocally confirmed. But in view of other data, it seems plausible that it will become possible to identify normal apoB genes associated with increased risk for myocardial infarction.

We have searched for variability gene effects at the apoB locus and found deviations in mean within-pair difference in MZ twin pairs between two categories of homozygotes in an RFLP detectable with the restriction

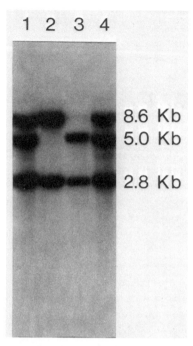

Figure 1-2 XbaI restriction site polymorphism at the apoB locus, corresponding to the third base of the codon for amino acid 2,488 in the mature protein. A Southern blot with DNA from four individuals (1–4) is shown. The polymorphism reflects an XbaI site that if present causes an 8.6 kilobase (kb) fragment to be split into a 5.0 kb fragment which is detected with the probe used, and a 3.6 kb fragment which is not detected (the 2.8 kb fragment is constant and does not belong to the polymorphism). Person 3 is homozygous for presence of the restriction site and exhibits no 8.6 kb fragment, only the 5.0 kb fragment, whereas person 2 is homozygous for absence of the restriction site and has only 8.6 kb fragment, no 5.0 kb fragment. Persons 1 and 4 are heterozygotes and have both fragments.

endonuclease EcoRI, corresponding to amino acid 4,154 in the mature protein. This polymorphism reflects an amino acid substitution and could therefore cause structural changes to apoB (Table 1-9). The EcoRI polymorphism is in strong linkage disequilibrium with a 3′ flanking hypervariable region (Berg, 1990c). The latter polymorphism reflects varying numbers of a 15 (or 2 × 15) base pair repeat in the 3′ flanking area. Scoring only 3 "genes", highly significant differences in within-pair variation in apoB levels were found between MZ twin pairs of two different categories of homozygotes (Table 1-9). Although this must be interpreted with caution, it is noteworthy that the association between each polymorphism and amount of within-pair variance was in agreement with the association between the two polymorphisms themselves.

There is a less strong allelic association between the XbaI polymorphism and the EcoRI polymorphism at the apoB locus, so not detecting the

Table 1-9 Mean within-pair difference in age and sex adjusted apolipoprotein B level (ΔapoB) in healthy Norwegian MZ twin pairs homozygous in an EcoRI restriction site polymorphism (2 alleles) at the apoB locus corresponding to amino acid 4,154 in mature apoB, or in a polymorphism (3 alleles scored) reflecting varying numbers of a 30 (2 × 15) base pair repeat in the 3′ flanking area of the apoB gene*

Homozygous genotype	Polymorphism detectable with EcoRI		Polymorphism in hypervariable 3′ flanking region	
	No. of pairs	ΔapoB (mg/dl)	No. of pairs	ΔapoB (mg/dl)
1–1	104	8.7[a]	2	1.4
2–2	5	16.8[a]	84	8.1[b]
3–3	—	—	7	14.7[b]

* Adapted from Berg (1990c).
[a] t = 2.47, p = 0.02.
[b] t = 2.53, p = 0.01.

above variability gene effect with the XbaI polymorphism does not detract from the importance of the suggested variability gene effect detected with the two polymorphisms discussed above. Interestingly, Tikkanen et al. (1990) recently reported differences between people possessing and people lacking the XbaI restriction site with respect to total, LDL, and HDL cholesterol, as well as apoB and response to diet intervention. The greater response was observed in people possessing the XbaI restriction site. At face value these data appear to confirm our indications that variability gene effects reside in the apoB gene with respect to lipid and apolipoprotein levels. Our own data would be best compatible with such an effect residing in the 3′ part of the gene. There is a need for more research.

The genes contributing to a different CAD risk factor, obesity, are not known. Rajput-Williams et al. (1988) found that certain haplotypes reflecting closely linked RFLPs at the apoB locus were associated with obesity, and LDL allotypes reflecting genetic apoB variation appear to be associated with leanness or fatness in swine (personal communication from Dr. Jan Rapacz). In our own studies of healthy people we have not yet seen convincing level gene effects with respect to body mass index. We have searched for variability gene effects with respect to body mass index at apolipoprotein loci, and obtained suggestive evidence for such an effect at the apoB locus. In the allotypic Ag system of LDL, sex and age adjusted within-pair difference in body mass index was significantly lower in MZ twin pairs of phenotype Ag(x+) than in MZ pairs with phenotype Ag (x−) (Berg, 1990d). In the EcoRI polymorphism corresponding to amino acid 4,154 in mature apoB, we found that MZ twin pairs who were homozygous for absence of the restriction site had a higher within-pair difference in body mass index than did pairs who were homozygous for presence of the site (Berg, 1990d). As mentioned above, this EcoRI polymorphism is

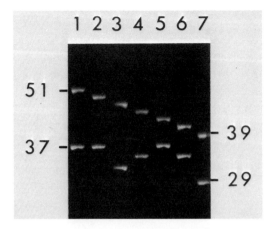

Figure 1-3 Polymerase chain reaction (PCR) products reflecting a polymorphism caused by varying numbers of a 15 base pair (bp) repeat (detected as a 2 × 15 bp repeats) in the 3' flanking area of the apoB gene. DNA from seven individuals (1–7) were submitted to amplification of the relevant area, by the PCR technique and the products were submitted to electrophoresis. Eleven different "alleles" are visualized, but more are known to exist. The numbers 29, 37, 39, and 51 indicate number of 15 bp repeats in "allele."

relatively close to the polymorphism of the hypervariable region in the 3' flanking area of the apoB gene. Variability gene effect seems to exist also for this polymorphism, but there is a need to repeat the studies with techniques that can distinguish many more genes than the Southern blot techniques used in the above studies (See Fig. 1-3). We tentatively conclude that the 3' part of the apoB gene may influence variability of quantitative lipoprotein parameters as well as body mass index.

DNA Variation at the ApoC-II Locus

Our studies have yielded evidence suggestive of variability gene effect on age and sex adjusted fasting triglycerides by a BglI polymorphism at the apolipoprotein C-II locus, but more studies are needed.

Genetic Variation at Lipase Loci

Reports on attempts to uncover correlation between genetic variation at lipase loci and lipid levels or CAD are beginning to appear. One group of workers found association between triglyceride level and DNA variants at the lipoprotein lipase locus (Chamberlain et al., 1989). Although confirmation is needed, there is little doubt that the lipase genes are another set of interesting candidate genes to study.

Normal DNA Variation at the Locus for Cholesteryl Ester Transfer Protein (CETP)

Reverse cholesterol transport is the least examined and least understood part of lipid metabolism. Since extrahepatic tissues lack the capacity to degrade sterols to the excretable form of bile acids, excess cholesterol in such tissues must be transported by the plasma to the liver for catabolism. Reverse cholesterol transport (Fielding and Fielding, 1982) involves several reactions including transfer of cholesteryl esters to serum lipoproteins by cholesteryl ester transfer proteins (CETPs). Although several groups of workers have reported proteins active in cholesteryl ester transfer between plasma lipoprotein particles and (presumably) between cells and plasma lipoproteins, the highly active CETP described by Jarnagin et al. (1987) may represent the functional component of previous preparations. Drayna et al. (1987) have cloned and sequenced CETP cDNA, and RFLPS in DNA at the CETP locus have been detected (Drayna and Lawn, 1987).

Variation in efficiency of removing cholesteryl esters from tissues for transport to the liver or of cholesteryl ester transfer between lipoprotein classes could be of importance for susceptibility or resistance to atherosclerosis. Accordingly, the CETP locus is a candidate locus with respect to atherosclerosis. We have examined the relationship between DNA variants (in the TaqI "B" polymorphism) at this locus and established CAD risk factors or protective factors (Kondo et al., 1989). We observed a statistically significant level gene effect on apoA-I concentration and to a certain extent on HDL cholesterol concentration (Table 1-10).

The effect of CETP genotype on apoA-I and HDL cholesterol was only present in nonsmokers (Kondo et al., 1989). Thus, smokers do not have the potential advantage of an increased apoA-I level had by nonsmokers who are homozygous for the 2-allele in the TaqI "B" polymorphism at the

Table 1-10 Sex and age adjusted HDL cholesterol and apoA-I levels in people of different genotypes in the TaqI "B" polymorphism in DNA at the CETP locus*

Genotype	No. of persons	HDL cholesterol (mmol/l)		ApoA-I (mg/dl)	
		Mean	SD	Mean	SD
1–1	46	1.27	0.35	139[a]	22
1–2	76	1.39	0.36	147[b]	22
2–2	24	1.48[c]	0.44	158	33
Total	146	1.37	0.37	146	25

* Adapted from Kondo et al. (1989).
[a] Significance of difference from 2-2 group: p = 0.005 (p = 0.005 if log10 values are used).
[b] Significance of difference from 2-2 group: p = 0.05 (p = 0.065 if log10 values are used).
[c] Significance of difference from 1-1 group: p = 0.03 (p = 0.04 if log10 values are used).

CETP locus. This is an interesting illustration of interaction between environmental and genetic factors in determining the level of a CAD risk or protective factor (see Introduction).

Summary

Studies of DNA variation at CAD candidate loci have not yet led to the detection of markers that without any doubt are strong predictors of CAD. However, interesting level gene effects have been uncovered, together with important suggestions of variability gene effects, and gene-environment interactions.

GENE-GENE INTERACTION AND CAD RISK FACTORS

It is likely that many of the genetically influenced risk factors such as high cholesterol level are influenced by several genes, and gene-gene interaction is likely to be important in determining CAD risk. Recently, the first example of interaction between normal genes in determining CAD risk factor variation was reported.

Pedersen and Berg (1988, 1990), in two independent series found that normal variation at the LDLR locus expressed as a PvuII restriction site polymorphism that is apparently in linkage disequilibrium with functionally important domains, is associated with total and LDL cholesterol levels. This finding has been confirmed by other workers. This observation extended the clinical importance of variation at the LDLR locus far beyond that of the rare autosomal dominant hypercholesterolemia.

When people were divided according to presence or absence of the apoE4 isoform, which is known to significantly increase cholesterol level, it turned out that this effect was present only in people who lacked the PvuII restriction site (Table 1-11). The data in Table 1-11 are those from

Table 1-11 Interaction between apoE alleles and normal alleles at the LDLR locus expressed as a PvuII restriction site polymorphism, in determining age and sex adjusted total cholesterol*

| ApoE4 allele | Mean total cholesterol (mmol/l) in people with LDLR genotype | | |
	A2A2	A1A1 or A1A2	In total series
Present	7.06^a (n = 31)	5.87 (n = 15)	6.67 (n = 46)
Absent	6.08^a (n = 69)	5.84 (n = 41)	5.99 (n = 110)

* Adapted from Pedersen and Berg (1989).

^{a} t = 3.90, p < 0.001.

(n = number).

the first series examined. In the total series, mean sex and age adjusted total cholesterol was 6.67 mmol/l in people possessing and 5.99 mmol/l in people lacking the apoE4 allele. In people lacking the PvuII restriction site at the LDLR locus (genotype A2A2), the difference between those having and those lacking the apoE4 allele in total cholesterol was 1 mmol/l (see Table 1-11) whereas there was no difference between people with or without the apoE4 allele in those possessing the PvuII restriction site at their LDLR locus. Thus, a normal gene identified by the PvuII restriction site polymorphism totally abolished the strong effect of the apoE4 gene on cholesterol.

The discovery of the LDLR gene and apoE gene interaction in determining CAD risk factor level should stimulate the search for more gene-gene interactions. Until now, no example of interaction between variability genes appears to be known. It seems likely, however, that such gene-gene interactions will also be detected.

ECOGENETICS OF HUMAN ATHEROSCLEROSIS

Ecogenetics is the study of heritable variations in response to environmental agents including nutritional or lifestyle factors. Ecogenetics may be a useful concept in relation to human atherosclerosis and it may help to avoid exogenous factors being considered to the exclusion of genetic determinants, or *vice versa* (Berg, 1987a).

The existing evidence which shows that environmental as well as genetic factors contribute to atherosclerosis development and CAD must mean that environmental, nutritional, or lifestyle factors preferably cause disease in people who have a genetic predisposition. The genetic factors are only rarely of such strength that disease is almost inescapable, such as in some of the monogenic hyperlipidemias. Apparently, in most CAD cases, genes and lifestyle factors interact to produce atherosclerosis. Each single gene may not have a strong effect, but together with other genes shift the risk profile in an unfavorable direction if not counteracted by still other genes or by environmental factors. There are, however, also strong single-gene determinants of CAD risk other than the genes for hyperlipidemias. The gene(s) causing a high Lp(a) lipoprotein level is a good example of this. Those who preferentially contract early CAD presumably have an unfortunate combination of atherogenic genes and lifestyle factors.

We know from the significant decrease in CAD frequency in occupied European countries during World War II (see above) that even those with a genetic predisposition to atherosclerosis may escape disease for at least several years if lifestyle factors are changed in an antiatherogenic direction. This knowledge, together with a decline in myocardial infarction in several Western countries over the last decades, gives reason for cautious optimism that much may be achieved by introducing healthy diets and lifestyles.

Atherosclerotic diseases are common. Therefore, it is not surprising that genes which render the individual susceptible to atherosclerosis are common, such as genes belonging to normal polymorphisms. The analyses of normal genetic polymorphisms at candidate loci remain a strong research strategy to arrive at a better understanding of the ecogenetics of human atherosclerosis. The variability gene concept and the recent detection of gene-gene interaction in determining total and LDL cholesterol levels add important new dimensions to such studies.

ETHICAL, LEGAL, AND SOCIAL CONSEQUENCES OF PREDICTIVE TESTING FOR CAD RISK

There is little doubt that practically all genes contributing to atherosclerosis risk will be identified in the near future. The capability of predicting atherosclerosis risk should be used to improve disease prevention (see below) and to secure early diagnosis and treatment.

A compulsory CAD risk screening program would not be advisable because it would interfere with people's autonomy and may cause anxiety in inadequately informed people. It is important that people retain their freedom to act with respect to lifestyle. Such a freedom would be attenuated if screening were to be made mandatory. It appears that a system where predictive genetic screening is offered on a voluntary, fully informed basis and followed up with adequate counseling is the only one acceptable. For this to be effective, the public would have to be adequately educated. This would be a formidable task.

Even voluntary screening programs could, however, lead to unfavorable consequences for the individual, unless precautions are taken. Doubtless, a person could be hurt if it were to become known that she or he had a greatly increased risk to contract a serious disorder that could lead to early incapacitation or death. Accordingly, there is a strong need to protect the data originating from predictive genetic tests in a strict manner. It is our opinion that employers, prospective employers, life insurance companies, pension funds, educational institutions, the military, and other consumers of health data should be denied access to the results of predictive genetic tests on individuals. They should be forbidden to require that such tests be performed or to ask if predictive tests have been performed. Otherwise, unfortunate people would be discriminated against. Even in a system for voluntary testing there could be discrimination against the most responsible people (those who take the tests and assume responsibility for improved lifestyle and health) if test results are not fully protected from disclosure.

It should be kept in mind that with respect to frequent serious diseases such as atherosclerosis, the predisposing genes in the majority of cases are normal genes which by themselves do not necessarily lead to disease, but which alone or in concert with other genes increase a person's susceptibility to disease. Society has no established tradition yet for handling information on an individual's normal genes like those that communicate medical information about previous or current diseases to various consumers of health information. Results of predictive genetic tests should not be handled according to established practices for clinical information on manifest disease. The best protection would be laws making information about an individual's normal genes or genetic predisposition to common disorders the exclusive property of that individual. Only with strict data protection can the public trustfully make use of predictive genetic testing to prevent or delay the development of CAD.

Screening conducted early in life would make it possible to institute particularly efficient preventive efforts (e.g., from childhood on). It is plausible that the best results of preventive efforts may be expected when started at a young age. Furthermore, it is plausible that those people who from predictive genetic testing know that they have a particular risk, would be much more motivated than the population at large to make strong efforts at disease prevention. Thus, predictive genetic testing under the right circumstances holds considerable promise for more efficient disease prevention.

FAMILY ORIENTED PREVENTIVE MEDICINE

Even if one does not want to institute population-wide screening programs, genetic knowledge should be utilized in a setting of family oriented preventive medicine.

Elements of a program for family oriented preventive medicine should be activated whenever a person contracts CAD at a relatively young age: prior to ages 55–60 in males or 60–65 in females. It should also be instituted when there are other reasons to suspect genetic predisposition to CAD in a family. Examples of such reasons are the occurrence of early CAD in several second-degree or more distant relatives, several cases of sudden death in the family, or predictive testing that has indicated an increased risk.

A thorough family search for known genetic risk factors (predictive genetic testing in family) should be made and environmental risk factors should be recorded whenever a genetic predisposition to CAD is suspected. If risk factors are detected in some or all members of the nuclear family, rigorous preventive measures should be instituted in all members with risk factors, with the aim of reducing the levels of all risk factors that can be manipulated. In families where some (but not all) members have risk factors, all (also those without detectable risk factors) should be encouraged to participate in disease prevention efforts, so that disease prevention becomes a goal for the whole family.

In families where no genetic risk factor can be detected by methods available at present despite strong suspicion of disease susceptibility, rigorous preventive efforts should be instituted in all family members in order to achieve as low a level as possible of all risk factors that can be reduced.

The nuclear family should be used both as a motivating and an executing instrument for preventive efforts. It is likely that significant results can be achieved by family oriented preventive medicine (Berg, 1989b). Efforts at developing a family oriented preventive medicine should be accelerated and the results of such efforts carefully monitored.

REFERENCES

Armstrong, W.V., Cremer, P., Eberle, E., Manke, A., Schulze, F., Wieland, H., Kreuzer, H., and Seidel, D. (1986). *Atherosclerosis.* **62,** 249.

Aro, A. (1973) *Serum Lipids and Lipoproteins in First-Degree Relatives of Young Survivors of Myocardial Infarction.* Thesis, University of Helsinki.

Berg, K. (1963). *Acta Pathol. Microbiol. Scand.* **59,** 369.

Berg, K. (1964). *Acta Pathol. Microbiol. Scand.* **62,** 600.

Berg, K. (1968). *Ser. Haematol.* **1,** 111.

Berg, K. (1969). *Ann. NY. Acad. Sci.* **162,** 189.

Berg, K. (1971). In: *Proceedings of the IVth International Congress of Human Genetics Paris 1971.* Human Genetics, Excerpta Medica, Amsterdam. pp. 352–362.

Berg, K. (1979). In: *The Biochemistry of Atherosclerosis.* Scanu, A.M., Wissler, R.W., and Getz, G.S. (eds.). Marcel Dekker, Inc., New York. pp. 419–490.

Berg, K. (1981). In: *Twin Research 3: Part C, Epidemiological and Clinical Studies.* Gedda, L., Parisi, P., and Nance, W.E. (eds.). A.R. Liss, New York. pp 117–130.

Berg, K. (1983). In: *Progress in Medical Genetics* Vol. V. Steinberg, A.G., Bearn, A.G., Motulsky, A.G., and Childs, B. (eds.). W.B. Saunders Co., Philadelphia. pp. 35–90.

Berg, K. (1984). *Acta Genet. Med. Gemellol.* **33,** 349.

Berg, K. (1986). *Clin. Genet.* **30,** 515.

Berg, K. (1987a). In: *Atherosclerosis. Biology and Clinical Science.* Olsson, A.G. (ed.). Churchill-Livingstone, Edinburgh. pp. 323–337.

Berg, K. (1988). *Clin. Genet.* **33,** 102.

Berg, K. (1989a). *Amer. J. Clin. Nutr.* **49,** 1025.

Berg, K. (1989b). *Clin. Genet.* **36,** 299.

Berg, K. (1990a). In: *Lp(a) Lipoprotein. 25 Years of Progress.* Scanu, A. (ed.). Academic Press, San Diego. 1990.

Berg, K. (1990b). In: *From Phenotype to Gene in Common Disorders.* Berg, K., Retterstøl, N., and Refsum, S. (eds.). Munksgaard, Copenhagen. pp. 138–162.

Berg, K. (1990c). In: *From Phenotype to Gene in Common Disorders.* Berg, K., Retterstøl, N., and Refsum, S. (eds.). Munksgaard, Copenhagen. pp. 77–91.

Berg, K. (1990d). In: *Proceedings of the International Conference on Genetic Variation and Nutrition, Washington, June 22–23, 1989.* Simopoulos, A. (ed.). Karger, Basel. 1990.

Berg, K., Dahlén, G., and Børresen, A.-L. (1979). *Clin. Genet.* **16,** 347.

Berg, K., Dahlén, G., and Frick, M.H. (1974). *Clin. Genet.* **6,** 230.

Berg, K., Hames, C., Dahlén, G., Frick, M.H., and Krishan, I. (1976). *Proc. Natl. Acad. Sci. USA.* **73,** 937.

Berg, K., and Heiberg, A. (1976). In: *Birth Defects: Original Article Series,* XII. Bergsma, D. (ed.). pp. 266–270.

Berg, K., and Heiberg, A. (1977). In: *Birth Defects: Original Article Series,* XIV. Bergsma, D. (ed.). pp. 621–623.

Berg, K., Julsrud, J.O., Børresen, A.-L., Fey, G., and Humphries, S.E. (1984). *Cytogenet. Cell Genet.* **37,** 417.

Berg, K., Kondo, I., Drayna, D., and Lawn, R. (1990). *Clin. Genet.* **37,** 473.

Berg, K., and Leren, T.P. (1989). *Lancet* II, 812.

Berg, K., and Mohr, J. (1963). *Acta Genet.* **13,** 349.

Beynen, A.C., and Katan, M.B. (1985). *Atherosclerosis.* **57,** 19.

Brown, M.S., and Goldstein, J.L. (1974). *J. Biol. Chem.* **249,** 7306.

Brown, M.S., and Goldstein, J.L. (1976). *Science.* **191,** 150.

Brown, M.S., and Goldstein, J.L. (1986). *Science.* **232,** 34.

Brown, M.S., and Goldstein, J.L. (1987). *Nature.* **330,** 113.

Buraczynska, M., Hanzlik, J., and Grzywa, M. (1986). *Hum. Genet.* **74,** 165.

Børresen, A.L., Leren, T., Berg, K., and Solaas, M.H. (1987). *Hum. Hered.* **37,** 150.

Chamberlain, J.C., Thorn, J.A., Oka, K., Galton, D.J., and Stocks, J. (1989). *Atherosclerosis.* **79,** 85.

Dahlén, G. (1974). *Acta Med. Scand.* (suppl.), 570.

Dahlén, G., Berg, K., and Frick, M.H. (1976). *Clin. Genet.* **9,** 558.

Dahlén, G., Ericson, C., and Berg, K. (1978). *Clin. Genet.* **14,** 36.

Drayna, D.T., Hegele, R.A., Hass, P.E., Emi, M., Wu, L.L., Eaton, D.L., Lawn, R.M., Williams, R.R., White, R. L., and Lalouel, J.-M. (1988). *Genomics.* **3,** 230.

Drayna, D., Jarnagin, A.S., McLean, J., Henzel, W., Kohr, W., Fielding, C.J., and Lawn, R. (1987). *Nature.* **327,** 632.

Drayna, D., and Lawn, R. (1987). *Nucleic Acids Res.* **15,** 4698.

Durrington, P.N., Hunt, L., Ishola, M., Arrol, S., and Bhatnagar, D. (1988). *Lancet.* **i,** 1070.

Eaton, D.L., Fless, G.M., Kohr, W.J., McLean, J.W., Xu, Q.-T., Miller, C.G., Lawn, R.M., and Scanu, A.M. (1987). *Proc. Natl. Acad. Sci. USA.* **84,** 3224.

Elston, R.C., Namboodiri, K.K., Go, R.C.P., Siervogel, R.M., and Glueck, C.J. (1976). In: *Birth Defects. Original Article Series,* XII. Bergsma, D. (ed.). pp. 294–297.

Epstein, F.H. (1976). *Postgrad. Med.* **52,** 477.

Ferns, G.A.A., Ritchie, C., Satocks, J., and Galton, D.J. (1985). *Lancet* **ii,** 300.

Fielding, C.J., and Fielding, P.E. (1982). *Med. Clin. North Am.* **66,** 363.

Fless, G.M., Rolih, C.A., and Scanu, A.M. (1984). *J. Biol. Chem.* **259,** 1147.

Fless, G.M., ZumMallen, M.E., and Scanu, A.M. (1986). *J. Biol. Chem.* **261,** 8712.

Fogge, C.H. (1873). *Trans. Path. Soc.* **24,** 242.

Fredrickson, D.S., Levy, R.I., and Lees, R.S. (1967). *N. Engl. J. Med.* **276,** 32, 94, 148, 215, 273.

Frick, M.H., Dahlén, G., Berg, K., Valle, M., and Hekali, P. (1978). *Chest.* **73,** 62.

Friedlander, Y., Cohen, T., Stenhouse, N., Davis, A.M., and Stein, Y. (1982). *Isr. J. Med. Sci.* **18,** 1137.

Genest, J., Martin-Munley, S., McNamara, J.R., Salem, D.N., and Schaefer, E.J. (1989). *Circulation.* **80** (suppl. II), 180.

Glueck, C.J., Fallat, R., Buncher, C.R., Tsang, R., and Steiner, P. (1973). *Metabolism.* **22**, 1403.

Goldstein, J.L., and Brown, M.S. (1973). *Proc. Natl. Acad. Sci. USA.* **70**, 2804.

Goldstein, J.L., Hazzard, W.R., Schrott, H.G., Bierman, E.L., and Motulsky, A.G. (1972). *Trans. Assoc. Am. Physicians.* **85**, 120.

Groover, M.E., Jernigan, J.A., and Martin, C.D. (1960). *Am. J. Med. Sci.* **53**, 27.

Gurakar, A., Hoeg, J.M., Kostner, G., Papadopoulos, N.M., and Brewer, H.B. (1985). *Atherosclerosis.* **57**, 293.

Hajjar, K.A., Gavish, D., Breslow, J.L., and Nachman, R.L. (1989). *Nature.* **339**, 303.

Harpel, P.C., Gordon, B.R., and Parker, T.S. (1989). *Proc. Natl. Acad. Sci. USA.* **86**, 3847.

Hegele, R.A., et al. (1986). *N.Engl. J. Med.* **315**, 1509.

Heiberg, A. (1975). *Genetic and Clinical Studies of Hyperlipoproteinaemia in Xanthomatosis.* Thesis, University of Oslo.

Heiberg, A., and Berg, K. (1974). *Clin. Genet.* **5**, 144.

Heiberg, A., and Berg, K. (1976). *Clin. Genet.* **9**, 203.

Heyden, S., Heyman, A., and Camplong, L. (1969). *J. Chronic. Dis.* **22**, 105.

Hobbs, H.H., Leitersdorf, E., Leffert, C.C., Cryer, D.R., Brown, M.S., and Goldstein, J.L. (1989). *J. Clin. Invest.* **84**, 656.

Hofmann, S.L., Eaton, D.L., Brown, M.S., McConathy, W.J., Goldstein, J.L., and Hammer, R.E. (1990). *J. Clin. Invest.* **85**, 1542.

Jarnagin, A.S., Kohr, W., and Fielding, C.J. (1987). *Proc. Natl. Acad. Sci. USA.* **84**, 1854.

Jürgens, G., Ashy, A., and Zenker, G. (1989). *Lancet.* **i**, 911.

Karathanasis, S.K., Norum, R.A., Zannis, V.I., and Breslow, J.L. (1983a). *Nature.* **301**, 718.

Karathanasis, S.K., McPherson, J., Zannis, V.I., and Breslow, J.L. (1983b). *Nature.* **304**, 371.

Katan, M.B., Beynen, A.C., De Vries, J.H.M., and Nobels, A. (1986). *Am. J. Epidemiol.* **123**, 221.

Katan, M.B., and Beynen, A.C. (1987). *Am. J. Epidemiol.* **125**, 387.

Kessling, A.M., Horsthemke, B., and Humphries, S.E. (1985). *Clin. Genet.* **28**, 296.

Kessling, A.M., Berg, K., Møkleby, E., and Humphries, S.E. (1986). *Clin. Genet.* **29**, 485.

Kondo, I., and Berg, K. (1990). *Clin. Genet.* **37**, 132.

Kondo, I., Berg, K., Drayna, D., and Lawn, R. (1989). *Clin. Genet.* **35**, 49.

Law, A., Powell, L.M., Brunt, H., Knott, T.J., Altman, D.G., Rajput, J., Wallis, S.C., Pease, R.J., Priestley, L.M., Scott, J., Miller, G.J., and Miller, N.E. (1986). *Lancet* **i**, 1301.

Maartmann-Moe, K., and Berg, K. (1981). *Clin. Genet.* **20**, 352.

Maartmann-Moe, K., Magnus, P., Golden, W., and Berg, K. (1981a). *Clin. Genet.* **20**, 113.

Maartmann-Moe, K., Magnus, P., Børresen, A.-L., and Berg, K. (1981b). *Clin. Genet.* **20**, 337.

Magnus, P., Berg, K., Børresen, A.L., and Nance, W.E. (1981a). *Clin. Genet.* **19**, 67.

Magnus, P., Maartmann-Moe, K., Golden, W., Nance, W.E., and Berg, K. (1981b). *Clin. Genet.* **20,** 104.

Mayo, O., Fraser, G.R., and Stamatoyannopoulos, G. (1969). *Hum. Hered.* **19,** 86.

Mayo, O., Wiesenfeld, S.L., Stamatoyannopoulos, G., and Fraser, G.R. (1971). *Lancet* **ii,** 554.

McLean, J.W., Tomlinson, J.E., Kuang, W.-J., Eaton, D.L., Chen, E.Y., Fless, G.M., Scanu, A.M., and Lawn, R.M. (1987). *Nature.* **330,** 132.

Miles, L.A., Fless, G.M., Levin, E.G., Scanu, A.M., and Plow, E.F. (1989). *Nature.* **339,** 301.

Morris, S.W., and Price, W.H. (1985). *Lancet* **ii,** 1127.

Morton, N.E., Berg, K., Dahlén, G., Ferrell, R.E., and Rhoads, G.G. (1985). *Genet. Epidemiol.* **2,** 113.

Motulsky, A.G. (1976). *N. Engl. J. Med.* **294,** 823.

Müller, C. (1939). *Arch. Intern. Med.* **64,** 675.

Murray, J.C., Buetow, K.H., Donovan, M., Hornung, S., Motulsky, A.G., Disteche, C., Dyer, K., Swisshelm, K., Anderson, J., Giblett, E., Sadler, E., Eddy, R., and Shows, T.B. (1987). *Am. J. Hum. Genet.* **40,** 338.

Murray, J.C., Sadler, E., Eddy, R.L., Shows, T.B., and Buetow, K.H. (1985). *Cytogenet. Cell Genet.* **40,** 709.

Neven, L., Khalil, A., Pfaffinger, D., Fless, G.M., Jackson, E., and Scanu, A.M. (1990). *J. Lipid Res.* **31,** 633.

Nikkilä, E.A., and Aro, A. (1973). *Lancet* **1,** 954.

Nora, J.J., Lortscher, R.H., Spangler, R.D., Nora, A.H., and Kimberling, W.J. (1980). *Circulation.* **61,** 503.

Ordovas, J.M., Schaefer, E.J., Salem, D., Ward, R.H., Glueck, C.J., Vergani, C., Wilson, P.W.F., and Karathanasis, S.K. (1986). *N. Engl. J. Med.* **314,** 671.

Osler, W. (1897). *Lectures on Angina Pectoris and Allied States.* D. Appleton & Co., New York.

Ott, J., Schrott, H.G., Goldstein, J.L., Hazzard, W.R., Allen Jr., F.H., Falk, C.T., and Motulsky, A.G. (1974). *Am. J. Hum. Genet.* **26,** 598.

Pedersen, J., and Berg, K. (1988). *Clin. Genet.* **34,** 306.

Pedersen, J., and Berg, K. (1990). In: *From Phenotype to Gene in Common Disorders.* Berg, K., Retterstøl, N., and Refsum, S. (eds.). Munksgaard, Copenhagen. In press.

Price, W.H., Morris, S.W., Burgon, R., Donald, P.M., and Kitchin, A.H. (1986). *Lancet* **ii,** 1041.

Rajput-Williams, J., Wallis, S.C., Yarnell, J., Bell, G.I., Knott, T. J., Sweetnam, P., Cox, N., Miller, N.E., and Scott, J. (1988). *Lancet* **ii,** 1442.

Rath, M., Niendorf, A., Reblin, T., Dietel, M., Krebber, H.-J., and Beisiegel, U. (1989). *Arteriosclerosis.* **9,** 579.

Rees, A., Stocks, J., Paul, H., Ohuchi, Y., and Galton, D. (1986). *Hum. Genet.* **72,** 168.

Rees, A., Stocks, J., Sharpe, C.R., Vella, M.A., Shoulders, C.C., Katz, J., Jowett, N.I., Baralle, F.E., and Galton, D.J. (1985). *J. Clin. Invest.* **76,** 1090.

Rees, A., Stocks, J., Shoulders, C.C., Galton, D.J., and Baralle, F.E. (1983). *Lancet* **i,** 444.

Rhoads, G.G., Dahlén, G., Berg, K., Morton, N.E., and Dannenberg, A.L. (1986). *JAMA.* **256,** 2540.

Rider, A.K., Levy, R., and Fredrickson, D.S. (1970). *Circulation.* **41–42** (suppl. 3), 10.

Rissanen, A.M. (1979a). *Am. J. Cardiol.* **44**, 60.

Rissanen, A.M. (1979b). *Br. Heart J.* **42**, 294.

Rissanen, A.M., and Nikkilä, E.A. (1977). *Br. Heart J.* **39**, 875.

Rissanen, A.M., and Nikkilä, E.A. (1979). *Br. Heart J.* **42**, 373.

Rittner, C. (1971). *Vox Sang.* **20**, 526.

Rose, G. (1964). *Br. J. Prev. Soc. Med.* **18**, 75.

Rosenman, R.H., Brand, R.J., Jenkins, C.D., Friedman, M., Strans, R., and Wurm, M. (1975). *JAMA.* **233**, 872.

Schultz, J.S., Shreffler, D.C., and Sing, C.F. (1974). *Ann. Hum. Genet.* **38**, 39.

Shoulders, C.C., Ball, M.J., Mann, J.I., and Baralle, F.E. (1986). *Lancet.* **ii**, 1286.

Sing, C.F., Schultz, J.S., and Shreffler, D.C. (1974). *Ann. Hum. Genet.* **38**, 47.

Sing, C.R., and Orr, J.D. (1976). *Am. J. Hum. Genet.* **28**, 453.

Slack, J., and Evans, K.A. (1966). *J. Med. Genet.* **3**, 239.

Snowden, C.B., McNamara, P.M., Garrison, R.J., Feinleib, M., Kannel, W.B., and Epstein, F.H. (1982). *Am. J. Epidemiol.* **115**, 217.

Stunkard, A.J., Sorensen, T.I.A., Hanis, C., Teasdale, T.W., Chakraborty, R., Schull, W.J., and Schulsinger, F., (1986). *N. Engl. J. Med.* **314**, 193.

Swisshelm, K., Dyer, K., Sadler, F., and Disteche, C. (1985). *Cytogenet. Cell Genet.* **40**, 756.

Talmud, P., and Humphries, S. (1986). *Lancet* **ii**, 104.

Tikkanen, M.J., Xu, C.-F., Hämäläinen, T., Talmud, P., Sarna, S., Huttunen, J.K., Pietinen, P., and Humphries, S. (1990). *Clin. Genet.* **37**, 327.

Utermann, G., Duba, C., and Menzel, H. (1988a). *Hum. Genet.* **78**, 47.

Utermann, G., Kraft, H.-G., Menzel, H., Hopferwieser, T., and Seitz, C. (1988b). *Hum. Genet.* **78**, 41.

Utermann, G., Menzel, H.J., Kraft, H.G., Duba, H.C., Kemmier, H.G., and Seitz, C. (1987). *J. Clin. Invest.* **80**, 458.

Utermann, G., Pruin, N., and Steinmetz, A. (1979). *Clin. Genet.* **15**, 63.

Vella, M., Kessling, A., Jowett, N., Rees, A., Stocks, J., Wallis, S., and Galton, D. (1985). *Hum. Genet.* **69**, 275.

Walton, K.W. (1972). In: *Protides of the Biological Fluids,* 19th Colloquium 1971. Peeters, H. (ed.). Pergamon Press, Oxford. pp. 225–226.

Weitkamp, L.R., Guttormsen, S.A., and Schultz, J.S. (1988). *Hum. Genet.* **79**, 80.

Whitehead, A.S., Solomon, E., Chambers, S., Bodmer, W.F., Povey, S., and Fey, G. (1982). *Proc. Natl. Acad. Sci. USA.* **79**, 5021.

Williams, R.R. (1984). In: *Genetic Epidemiology of Coronary Heart Disease: Past, Present, Future.* Alan R. Liss, New York. pp. 89–91.

Williams, R.R., Dadone, M.M., Hunt, S.C., Jorde, L.B., Hopkins, P.N., Smith, J.B., Owen Ash, K., and Kuida, K. (1984). In: *Genetic Epidemiology of Coronary Heart Disease: Past, Present, Future.* Alan R. Liss, New York. pp. 419–442.

Williams, R.R., Hunt, S.C., Hopkins, P.N., Stults, B.M., Wu, L.L., Hasstedt, S.J., Barlow, G.K., Stephenson, S.H., Lalouel, J.-M., and Kuida, H. (1988). *JAMA.* **259**, 3579.

Yater, W.M., Traum, A.H., Brown, W.G., Fitzgerald, R.P., Geisler, M.A., and Wilcox, B.B. (1948). *Am. Heart J.* **36**, 334.

2

Hypertension

Hypertension is a major risk factor in atherosclerosis, heart disease, hemorrhagic and nonhemorrhagic stroke, and a principal cause of morbidity and mortality in developed nations throughout the world. In atherosclerosis, hypertension contributes to intimal injury and permeability in the interactive process of lipoprotein uptake and plaque formation. In the etiology of hemorrhagic stroke (excluding ruptured congenital aneurysms), the pathogenesis is likely to be rupture of microaneurysms resulting from arterionecrosis, which is characterized by infiltration into the intima of blood plasma with fibrin deposition, histolysis of the internal elastic lamina, and loss of medial smooth muscle cells.

In the United States, almost 58 million people have high blood pressure, which is more common in black Americans (38% are hypertensive) than in whites (29%). Japan (Ueshima et al., 1980) and China (Li et al., 1985) have high morbidity and mortality from hypertension and stroke, but lower risks of coronary artery disease than in the United States and Europe. In other populations, especially in nonindustrialized societies such as the Tokelau, the condition is rare, but blood pressure levels may then be adversely influenced by migration and changes in weight, diet, exercise, and social factors. Thus, differences may be explained by genetic factors, environmental factors, or a genetic-environmental interaction. Advances in the management of hypertension make the search for specific causes of this disease important so that appropriate preventive and therapeutic measures may be undertaken in a timely fashion. In 1972, the United States government launched a blood pressure awareness program. Since then, the annual rate of fatal strokes has been cut in half by identifying patients at risk and undertaking needed programs of prevention and treatment. In the same time frame the rate of fatal heart attacks has dropped by 34%—for a variety of reasons, including the assault on high blood pressure.

Blood pressure is a continuously distributed metric trait the maintenance of which depends on the complex interaction of baroreceptors, renal transport systems for sodium and potassium, blood volume, vasoactive peptides, various hormones, myocardial contractility, vascular resistance, and the central and autonomic nervous systems. High blood pressure occurs as a primary condition (essential hypertension) or as a manifestation of many known diseases, including a number of mendelizing conditions (some of which are mentioned elsewhere in this volume). Renal disease is the most common etiologic basis of secondary hypertension and may be subdivided into dozens of conditions ranging from the various forms of nephritis and renal vascular disease, through connective tissue disorders, to dominant and recessive types of polycystic kidneys. Then there are nonrenal causes, such as pheochromocytoma, coarctation of the aorta (hypertension of the upper body), primary aldosteronism, central nervous system disorders, eclampsia, and Cushing syndrome. However, the focus of this chapter will be on that type of high blood pressure that is not secondary to another disease, is not part of a mendelian syndrome, and usually has its peak onset in mid life. Stroke may have a familial basis apart from hypertension, such as berry aneurysm, arteriovenous fistula, and homocystinemia. Serum cholesterol, a major risk factor in coronary artery disease, does not appear to be a risk factor in stroke, and may even be inversely related (Iso et al., 1989).

The primary cause of essential hypertension continues to be a subject of debate. Major genes have been postulated as its cause; so have the cumulative effects of multiple genetic and environmental factors, each of which contribute a small amount to the phenotype. Progress has been made in defining the role of specific elements such as the renin-angiotensin system, the vascular wall, aldosterone, the kinins, prostaglandins, neurotransmitters, and baroreceptors in the regulation of blood pressure (Unger and Gohlke, 1990).

It will probably be possible in the near future to divide the category of essential hypertension into several etiologic subgroups, as well as to identify various syndromes in which essential hypertension is a prominent component. One such recently described new syndrome is familial dyslipidemic hypertension (Williams et al., 1988).

One has to start with a definition of hypertension. The problem of how to handle numbers that are continuously distributed and are subject to modest measurement error will not be solved here. Most investigators accept 140/90 as the beginning of high blood pressure in adults age 18 and older. The *1988 Report of the Joint Committee on Detection, Evaluation, and Treatment of High Blood Pressure* adheres to this standard (see References). Anything below this is generally accepted as "normal." There are data to support the idea that when adult blood pressure exceeds a level of 120/80, the risk of cardiovascular disease begins to increase. The *1988 Report* lists a diastolic pressure of less than 85 as normal and 85–89 as "high normal." If the diastolic pressure is less than 90, and the systolic pressure is over 140, the term isolated systolic hypertension is used.

The higher the pressure, the greater the risk of stroke, coronary artery disease, and heart disease: 180/120 represents more risk than 160/100, which in turn is a more serious risk factor than 140/90. Blood pressure has a tendency to increase with age. Certainly this is evident throughout childhood and is associated with growth (see Fig. 2-1). Whether or not the magnitude of increase in childhood is inevitable may be arguable. The progressive increase in blood pressure in adult life among Americans,

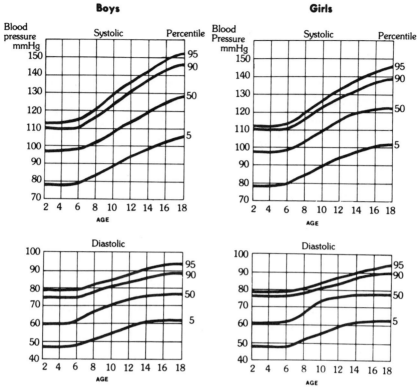

Figure 2-1 Increase in blood pressure during childhood with increasing age and growth.

Europeans, and Japanese is not the universal experience in certain other cultures. An important problem in the United States is hypertension among blacks, however, West Africans remaining in Africa do not share this problem.

GENETIC FACTORS

Although Morgagni, in 1769, apparently was the first to appreciate the familial nature of any cardiovascular disease in his report on strokes, genetic studies of hypertension did not advance steadily from this initial impetus. Early twin studies (Verschuer and Zipperlin, 1929; Stocks, 1930) revealed less variation in blood pressure among monozygotic (MZ) than dizygotic (DZ) twins. Platt (1963) reported severe hypertension in three sets of MZ twins. Family studies by several groups (Weitz, 1923; Ayman, 1934; Ostfeld and Paul, 1963) have compared recurrence risks for hypertension in families ascertained through a hypertensive member. Family studies, twin studies, and adoption studies (Borhani et al., 1976; Feinlieb and Garrison, 1979; Havlik et al., 1979; Heiberg et al., 1981) have provided consistent evidence for familial aggregation of blood pressure levels as well as for hypertension. In the case of systolic blood pressure, parent-offspring regressions are about 0.12 to 0.34. Dizygotic twin correlations are about 0.25 for systolic pressure and 0.27 for diastolic. In MZ twin pairs, Berg (1989) has reported heritability (h^2) of 0.64 for systolic and 0.51 for diastolic blood pressure measured as within-pair correlation coefficients. Adoption studies (Biron et al., 1977; Annest et al., 1979) also show higher correlation between biologic than between adoptive relatives.

Pickering and Platt have been among the most active investigators into the genetics of essential hypertension and systemic arterial blood pressure. Pickering (1968) has applied an age- and sex-adjusted score to his own data and to the material of others, including that collected by Søbye (1948). He has found curves that have slight positive skewness (but are log-normal) for a "normal" population, relatives of "normals," and relatives of hypertensive probands. However, the curve for relatives of hypertensives is shifted to the right, much as is seen in the hypothetical curve we have drawn for type C families with congenital heart disease (see Fig. 4-1). Independent studies by Ostfeld and Paul (1963) are in agreement with Pickering's etiologic position regarding the multifactorial inheritance of blood pressure and hypertension.

Platt (1963) has argued that a major gene effect may cause essential hypertension as have Morrison and Morris (1960). In a later publication, multifactorial inheritance has been acknowledged by Platt (1964) as an alternative not eliminated by his data. For hypertension, as well as for other cardiovascular disease, we do not see that there must be a strict dichotomy between polygenes and major genes. Skewed curves may be log-normal or bimodal. The advantage of Morton's model (Morton et al., 1970) of multifactorial inheritance is that it accommodates major genes within a predominantly polygenic mode.

The Hamilton-Pickering study (Hamilton-Pickering et al., 1954) has suggested a quantitative resemblance between first-degree relatives of hypertensive patients, from which a coefficient of resemblance was developed. Miall and Oldham (1963) were able to extend these concepts to the population at large. The coefficient of resemblance has been taken as a measure of the size of the genetic component of blood pressure in both "normal" and hypertensive families.

A careful reading of Pickering (1968) reveals his acceptance of the possibility of some major gene effects. Platt (1964), on the other hand, concedes that polygenic determinants are not eliminated, and that the major gene effects relate to the "tendency" to develop high blood pressure. The dispute may boil down to the size of the population of hypertensives influenced by major genes, as opposed to those with elevated pressures on a normal distribution curve. Pickering would admit only a small number of major gene-influenced patients—Platt would have a considerably larger group.

ENVIRONMENTAL FACTORS

Salt (sodium) and stress are two environmental risk factors that have been studied in human populations (Dahl et al., 1954) and animal models. Many nonindustrialized societies exhibit a low prevalence of hypertension and little or no increase in blood pressure with age (Epstein and Eckoff, 1967). However, some populations (e.g., Japan) that have high-salt diets also have an unusually high prevalence of hypertension. With exposure to an industrialized culture, the distribution of blood pressure within the population may change (Cruz-Coke et al., 1973; Ward et al., 1980) due to a variety of possible reasons, including diet (increased sodium, decreased potassium), obesity, exercise deficiency, stress, socioeconomic factors, and medications (e.g., birth control hormones). Ethnic comparisons of the incidence of hypertension and the distribution of blood pressure with age, as well as migration studies in which changes in the distribution of blood pressure have been documented following the relocation of a population to a different environment lend support to the importance of environmental factors in the etiology of hypertension.

GENETIC-ENVIRONMENTAL INTERACTION

The term genetic-environmental interaction appears throughout this volume. One feature of this etiologic mode is that the phenotypic effects of a specific genotype may or may not be expressed depending on the environment—that is, individuals in a population may not respond in the same way to the same environmental stimulus.

Animal homologies have demonstrated that heterogeneity of hypertension and the role of genetic-environmental interaction in its etiology. There are some interesting strains of rats that give us ideas on what may go into producing high blood pressure in humans. First, there is a hereditary predisposition. Some rats are not salt sensitive and do not get hypertension even when fed large amounts of sodium, but ALR and SHR strains do (Dahl, 1962; Rapp and Iwai, 1976). So if a rat with unfavorable heredity is given salt and stress, the rat gets high blood pressure. In the SHR strain, the high blood pressure leads to stroke. In the ALR strain, the high blood pressure produces plaques in the blood vessels, similar to those found in humans that can also lead to heart attacks. Thus one strain gets strokes and the other gets more generalized hardening of the arteries. Other strains of rats can be subjected to salt and stress and not get high blood pressure or any other apparent adverse changes.

Approximately 60% of human adults with hypertension are salt-sensitive on the basis of salt-loading tests (Fujita et al., 1980). Heredity predisposition interacting with various environmental triggers is a reasonable way to look at high blood pressure and its consequences in many families. If those at high risk could be clearly identified, a preventive strategy could be devised.

To us, the most useful first step to identify individuals at increased risk of essential hypertension is the finding of a positive family history. In fact, we are reluctant to diagnose essential hypertension in a young person who does not have such a history—instead we first redouble our efforts to find a cause of secondary hypertension. For essential hypertension, tests such as salt-loads (Grim et al., 1979), measurements of the urinary excretion of vasoactive peptides, the kinetics of sodium-potassium (Poston et al., 1981) and sodium-lithium transport (Canessa et al., 1980), blood pressure responses to cold, pain, dynamic isometric exercise (Ohlsson and Henningsen, 1978), and mental stress have been employed (Falkner et al., 1979); Poston et al., 1981).

Although it is occasionally difficult to determine at an early age if a child will have high blood pressure at a later age, blood pressure tracks reasonably well, and for those individuals identified during childhood, it should be possible to begin lifestyle changes in diet physical activity, and stress management to prevent or substantially delay the development of the disease. Childhood obesity has emerged as a risk factor (Lauer and Clark, 1989). The heritability of body mass is 0.76 in Berg's (Berg, 1989) data. In the previously discussed animal models, hypertension is often permanently fixed before maturity, so there is some urgency to search for the child at risk. The offspring of hypertensive probands have been subjected to various provocative tests to identify individuals who may be predisposed to hypertension. In ongoing studies, cross-sectional samples of infants and children have been followed longitudinally to assess tracking (on the assumption that the same genes that affect blood pressure in the adult are also active in young children).

RECENT ADVANCES IN GENETIC EVALUATION

Restriction fragment length polymorphisms (RFLPs) provide a powerful new method of Genetic Evaluation. The cosegregation of specific genetic markers (RFLPs) with a trait of interest (i.e., hypertension) may be examined in linkage and association studies using maximum likelihood methods.

Partitioned twin analysis has been advocated by Nance (1984) as a valuable tool in cardiovascular research. Genes that determine the synthesis of angiotensin, aldosterone, renin, bradykinin, endothelium, and neural receptors of various types would be useful candidates for investigation. In this technique, twins and their parents are typed for highly polymorphic genetic markers (RFLPs) and the DZ pairs are classified into subsets and compared with MZ twins who not only share alleles at the marker locus, but are identical for all other genes as well.

GENETIC COUNSELING AND PREVENTION

Our approach to counseling is to talk of familial tendency to high blood pressure and the excellent results that have been obtained, since about 1972, through early control of risk factors by lifestyle and dietary measures and, when necessary, pharmacologic intervention in those having the disease or a positive family history. It is obvious that the most careful evaluation for various genetic causes of hypertension and stroke (discussed in other chapters) and underlying diseases (e.g., renal disease, coarctation of the aorta) must be undertaken before concluding that the appropriate diagnosis is essential hypertension and not secondary hypertension.

REFERENCES

Annest, J.L., Sing, C.F., Biron, P., and Mongeau, J.G. (1979). *Am. J. Epidemiol.* **110,** 492.

Ayman, D. (1934). *Arch Intern. Med.* **53,** 792.

Berg, K. (1989). *Am. J. Clin. Nutr.* **49,** 1025.

Biron, P., Mongeau, J.G., and Bertrand, D. (1977). *Epidemiology and Control of Hypertension.* Grune & Stratton, New York. pp. 397–405.

Borhani, N.O., Feinlieb, M., Garrison, R.J., Christian, J.C., and Rosenman, R.H. (1976). *Acta. Genet. Med. Gemellol.* **25,** 137.

Canessa, M., Adragna, N., Solomon, H.S., Connelly, T.M., and Tosterson, D.C. (1980). *N. Engl. J. Med.* **302,** 772.

Cruz-Coke, R., Donoso, H., and Barrera, R. (1973). *Clin. Sci. Mol. Med.* **45** (suppl. 1), 55s.

Dahl, L.K., Heine, M., and Tassinari, L. (1962). *J. Exp. Med.* **115,** 1173.

Dahl, L.K., and Love, R.A. (1954). *Arch. Intern. Med.* **94,** 525.

Epstein, F.H., and Eckoff, R.D. (1967). *The Epidemiology of Hypertension.* Grune & Stratton, New York. p. 155.

Falkner, B., Onesti, G., Angelakos, E.G., Fernandes, M., and Langman, C. (1979). *Hypertension* **1,** 23.

Feinlieb, M., and Garrison, R.J. (1979). *Genetic Analysis of Common Diseases.* A.R. Liss, New York. p. 653.

Fujita, T., Henry, W.L., Bartter, F.C., Lake, C.R., and Delea, C.S. (1980). *Kidney Int.* **21,** 371.

Grim, C.E., Luft, F.C., Miller, J.A., Brown, P.L., Gannon, M.A., and Weinberger, M.H. (1979). *J. Lab. Clin. Med.* **94,** 764.

Hamilton, M., Pickering, G.W., and Roberts, J.A.F. (1954). *Clin. Sci.* **13,** 11, 273.

Havlik, R.J., Garrison, R.J., Katz, S.H., Ellison, R.C., Feinlieb, M., and Myrianthopoulous, N.C. (1979). *Am. J. Epidemiol.* **109,** 512.

Heiberg, A., Magnus, P., Berg, K., and Nance, W.E. (1981). *Twin Research*. **3,** 163.

Iso, H., Jacobs, D.R., Wentworth, D., Neaton, J.D., and Cohen, J.D. (1989). *N. Engl. J. Med.* **320,** 904.

Lauer, R.M., and Clarke, W.R. (1989). *Pediatrics* **84,** 633.

Li, S.C., Schoenberg, B.S., Wang, C.C., Cheng, X.M., Bolis, C.L., and Wang, K.J. (1985). *Neurology* **35,** 1708.

Miall, W.E., and Oldham, P.D. (1963). *Br. Med. J.* **I,** 75.

Morgagni, J.B. (1769). *The Seats and Causes of Disease Investigated by Anatomy*.

Morrison, S., and Morris, J. (1960). *Lancet* **2,** 829.

Morton, N.E., Yee, S., and Elston, R.C. (1970). *Clin. Genet.* **1,** 81.

Nance, W.E. (1984). *Prog. Clin. Biol. Res.* **147,** 325.

1988 Report of the Joint National Committee on Detection, Evaluation, and Treatment of High Blood Pressure. (1988). NIH Publication No. 88-1088.

Ohlsson, O., and Henningsen, N.C. (1978). *Acta. Med. Scand.* **625** (suppl.), 7.

Ostfeld, A.M., and Paul, O. (1963). *Lancet* **1,** 575.

Pickering, G.W. (1968). *High Blood Pressure,* ed. 2. Churchill, London.

Platt, R. (1963). *Lancet* **1,** 899.

Platt, R. (1964). *Practitioner*. **193,** 5.

Poston, L., Sewell, R.B., Wilkinson, S.P., Richardson, P.J., Williams, R., Clarkson, E.M., MacGregor, G.A., and de Wardener, H.E. (1981). *Br. Med. J.* **282,** 847.

Rapp, J.P., and Iwai, J. (1976). *Clin. Exp. Pharmacol. Physiol.* **3** (suppl.), 11.

Søbye, P. (1948). *Op. Domo. Biol. Here. Hum. KbH,* 16.

Stocks, P. (1930). *Ann. Eugen.* **4,** 49.

Ueshima, H., et al. (1980). *Prev. Med.* **9,** 722.

Unger, T., and Gohlke, P. (1990). *Am. J. Cardiol.* **65,** 31.

Verschuer, O., and Zipperlin, V. (1929). *Z. Klin. Med.* **112,** 69.

Ward, R.H., Chin, P.G., and Prior, I.A.M. (1980). *Genetic Analysis of Common Diseases: Applications to Predictive Factors in Coronary Disease*. A.R. Liss, New York. p. 675.

Weitz, W. (1923). *Z. Klin. Med.* **96,** 151.

Williams, R.R., et al. (1988). *JAMA* **259,** 3579.

3

Rheumatic Fever

Although rheumatic fever (RF) is not currently a pressing topic in the genetics of cardiovascular disease, for the sake of completeness, we present a brief discussion of the cardiovascular disease that received the first attempt at systematic genetic analysis. The historical irony is that, of all the cardiovascular diseases, rheumatic fever turns out to be the one most dependent on an environmental trigger.

GENETIC-ENVIRONMENTAL INTERACTION

Cheadle (1889), in his Harveian lectures, first pointed out that rheumatic fever occurred in familial clusters. Certain racial and ethnic groups have also been singled out as being particularly susceptible to the disease. The Irish and Scandinavian immigrants in the United States were stigmatized as rheumatic fever-prone (Coburn, 1931; Stroud and Twaddle, 1950). In fact, red hair and freckles were for a short time considered to be sentinel findings in susceptible individuals, until the concept shifted to an ethnic explanation that so many of the rheumatic fever patients in Boston had red hair and freckles because the population had a large Irish component.

Many Scandinavian families in the midwestern United States, including the family of one of the authors (JJN), were devastated by rheumatic fever at the turn of the century. Yet in Scandinavian countries today, rheumatic fever has essentially been abolished. In Scandinavian-Americans in the Midwest, the disease has also been disappearing. However, there have been recent outbreaks in Ohio (Hosier et al., 1987). Sixty years ago, blacks were thought to be less susceptible than whites, but within the past 25 years it has been observed that urban blacks are afflicted more frequently than whites (Quinn et al., 1967). Hispanic populations in the United States and Mexico are also inordinately burdened by rheumatic fever. But there has also been a recent resurgence of RF among middle class whites in the western United States (Veasy et al., 1987).

In some instances, a socioeconomic explanation can be offered (Coburn, 1960). Reduction of poverty in certain susceptible populations appears to have greatly improved the attack rate. But where poverty has not been significantly reduced and where urban crowding has been added, the disease prevails. Populations that may have the same or may truly have less genetic susceptibility come to our attention because of the persistence of adverse environmental conditions. Socioeconomic factors may thus underlie part of the changing pattern of the disease. However, even before antibacterial therapy had any significant impact, a decrease in both the prevalence and severity of the disease was being recognized. It is thus possible to attribute a substantial portion of the decreased attack rate to improved living conditions, better hygiene, and prevention of recurrences.

The changing presentation over the previous three decades (dramatic decrease in the epistaxis and chorea) and severity (decrease in mortality, prolonged course, residual heart disease, and rheumatic pneumonia) may not be as readily explained. Alterations in the *beta-hemolytic streptococcus* and its capacity to induce different immune responses must be considered in the light of recent evidence of the deviant pathogenicity of the organism (Veasy et al., 1987; Stevens et al., 1989). The mucoid strains are possibly becoming more rheumatogenic after a quiescent period during which the organism had been less virulent. However, it still appears to be the poor who have the most florid clinical disease.

What is clear is that rheumatic fever is an everchanging disease, changing from worse to better to perhaps worse again. Antibacterial therapy has been a major force for change, and improved socioeconomic conditions have made a significant contribution. Ethnic and racial predisposition may exist, but is greatly curtailed by appropriate management of streptococcal infections.

It is obvious that discussion of ethnic predisposition has genetic implications. A review of the meager amount of literature of genetic studies of rheumatic fever starts with the work of Wilson and Schweitzer (1937). These authors looked at three possible explanations for the familial incidence of RF: common environment, communicability, and hereditary susceptibility. They successively rejected common environment and communicability (in the traditional sense of contagion). They then approached the disease as a heritable one and looked at autosomal recessive and dominant modes for single locus and two or more loci. They also analyzed for X-linked inheritance. The conclusion was that hereditary susceptibility to rheumatic fever was transmitted as an autosomal recessive trait. The authors hedged their bet by adding that heredity "may not necessarily be the sole condition essential for the development of the disease."

Wilson (Wilson et al., 1943; Wilson and Schweitzer, 1954), in subsequent publications, reinforced the hereditary position. For those trained after a consensus had been reached concerning the streptococcal role in the etiology of RF, it should be emphasized that there were many other knowledgeable cardiologists and rheumatologists who also took over twenty years to embrace the concept that the streptococcus was the environmental trigger in this disease (Coburn, 1931). There was confirmation of a genetic hypothesis from other sources (Mallen and Castillo, 1952; Gray et al., 1952). Stevenson and Cheeseman (1953, 1956) concluded that there were important genetic factors, but that these factors did not fit autosomal recessive inheritance.

Twin studies have been undertaken to investigate the genetic contribution. Taranta et al. (1959) found 19% concordance for rheumatic fever in monozygotic twin pairs and 5% concordance among dizygotic twins. This is consistent with expectation in multifactorial inheritance and is comparable to what has been found in congenital heart diseases (Nora et al., 1967). ABO blood groups, secretor status, and haptoglobins have been studied, but have not been as useful as one would hope.

To us, the most productive field for understanding both the pathogenesis of RF and the genetic predisposition is through immunologic and immunogenetic studies. The studies of Kaplan (Kaplan, 1960; Kaplan and Meyerserian, 1962; Kaplan et al., 1967) have provided a matrix for this understanding. This elegant work began with the concept of autoantibodies in rheumatic fever, proceeded through the demonstration of shared antigen between the *beta-hemolytic streptococcus* and cardiac tissue to definition of the properties of the cross reacting antigens.

Carrying this work one step further led to the investigation of the homologous leucocytic antibodies (HLA) antigens. Several rheumatic diseases, including juvenile rheumatoid arthritis and ankylosing spondylitis, have been found to have a strong association with class I or class II antigens. No class I antigen (HLA-A,B,C) relationship has proved to be informative, but at least three class II antigens have been suggested to show an association from different populations: DR-1 (Maharaj et al., 1987) and DR-2 (Ayoub et al., 1986) in blacks; and DR-4 in whites (Ayoub et al., 1986) and in Saudis (Rajapaske et al., 1987). Evidence has been put forward for an immunosuppressor susceptibility gene linked to HLA (Hafez et al., 1987) and for nonHLA B-cell antigens in RF patients (Khanna et al., 1989). The immunogenetic evaluation of rheumatic fever is underway, but is currently far from clear.

A summary statement on the genetics of rheumatic fever is that one should approach the subject as the genetics of susceptibility to rheumatic fever. A group A beta-hemolytic streptococcal infection of the respiratory tract is the essential trigger without which the disease would not occur. However, only about 0.3% of untreated group A streptococcal infections in an open population and 3% of untreated infections in a closed population (e.g., a military base) lead to rheumatic fever. These findings are compatible with an important genetic predisposition in the host. This predisposition may be monogenic or polygenic or both.

PREVENTION

Rheumatic fever recapitulates the etiologic considerations of the other major cardiovascular diseases. A genetic-environmental interaction underlies the disease. Both components may be studied with the intent of defining the patient at risk and eliminating the environmental trigger which produces the actual disease state. The ultimate goal in the etiologic study of all the cardiovascular diseases is prevention. Here, rheumatic fever may serve as a model because the means of prevention to the point of eradication has been defined. We now await only the aggressive implementation of these means.

REFERENCES

Ayoub, E.M., Barrett, D.J., Maclaren, N.K., and Krischer, J.P. (1986). *J. Clin. Invest.* **77,** 2019.

Cheadle, W.B. (1889). *Lancet* **1,** 821.

Coburn, A.F. (1960). *Am. J. Med. Sci.* **240,** 687.

Coburn, A.F. (1931). *The Factor of Infection in the Rheumatic State.* Williams & Wilkins, Baltimore.

Gray, F.G., Quinn, R.W., and Quinn, J.P. (1952). *Am. J. Med.* **13,** 400.

Hafez, M., el-Shennawy, F., el-Ziny, M., Abo-el-Hasan, S., and Khashaba, M. (1987). *Dis. Markers.* **5,** 177.

Hosier, D.M., Craenen, J.M., Teske, D.W., and Wheeler, J.J. (1987). *Am. J. Dis. Child.* **141,** 730.

Kaplan, M.H. (1960). *Ann. NY. Acad. Sci.* **86,** 974.

Kaplan, M.H., Espinoza, E., and Frengley, J.D. (1967). *Fed. Proc.* **26,** 701.

Kaplan, M.H., and Myerserian, M. (1962). *Lancet* **1,** 706.

Khanna, A.K., Buskirk, D.R., Williams, R.C., Gibofsky, A., Crow, M.K., Menon, A., Fotino, M., Reid, H.M., Poon-King, T., and Ribinstein, P. (1989). *J. Clin. Invest.* **83,** 1710.

Mallen, M.S., and Castillo, F. (1952). *Arch. Inst. Cardiol. Mex.* **22,** 136.

Maharaj, B., Hammond, M.G., Appadoo, B., Leary, W.P., and Pudifin, D.J. (1987). *Circulation.* **76,** 259.

Nora, J.J., Gilliland, J.C., and Sommerville, R.J. (1967). *N. Engl. J. Med.* **277,** 568.

Quinn, R.W., Downey, F.M., and Federspiel, C.F. (1967). *Public Health Rep.* **82,** 673.

Rajapakse, C.N., Halim, K., Al-Orainey, I., Al-Nozha, M., and Al-Aska, A.K. (1987). *Br. Heart J.* **58,** 659.

Stevens, D.L., Tanner, M.H., Winship, J., Swarts, R., Ries, K.M., Schlievert, P.M., Kaplan, E. (1989). *N. Engl. J. Med.* **321,** 1.

Stevenson, A.C., and Cheeseman, E.A. (1953). *Ann. Eugen. Lond.* **17,** 177.

Stevenson, A.C., and Cheeseman, E.A. (1956). *Ann. Hum. Genet.* **21,** 139.

Stroud, W.D., and Twaddle, P.H. (1950). *JAMA* **114,** 629.

Taranta, A., Torosdag, S., and Metrakos, J.D. (1959). *Circulation.* **20,** 778.

Veasy, L.G., Wiedmeier, S.E., and Orsmond, G.S. (1987). *N. Engl. J. Med.* **316,** 421.

Wilson, M.G., and Schweitzer, M.D. (1954). *Circulation.* **10,** 699.

Wilson, M.G., and Schweitzer, M.D. (1937). *J. Clin. Invest.* **14,** 555.

Wilson, M.G., Schweitzer, M.D., and Lubshez, R. (1943). *J. Pediatr.* **22,** 468, 581.

4

Congenital Heart Disease: Genetics

In this chapter we will present general concepts of the causes of familial congenital heart diseases, the genetic-environmental interaction, recurrence risks, and brief discussions of specific abnormalities. In chapters that follow, structural and functional abnormalities associated with environmental exposures, chromosomal anomalies, and single mutant genes will receive further attention.

In a monograph written on this subject (Nora and Nora, 1978b), we quoted Meister Eckhart who said "Only the hand that erases can write the truth." Each time we update the material on the causes of congenital heart disease (CHD) we find that considerable erasure is required. Not just for changes in tables, but changes in concepts. Doubtless, the erasures will continue over many years. For example, Table 4-1 is modified frequently, based on current evidence and criteria.

Although 5% of patients attending a congenital heart clinic have a chromosomal basis for their disease, this is a less meaningful figure than is the finding that about 10% of newborns with congenital heart disease have chromosomal anomalies (Hoffman and Christianson, 1978). Of course, case finding of congenital heart disease in patients with multiple abnormalities is different than case finding among otherwise normal infants with initially mild (and subtle) disease. Also, severely affected infants with trisomy 13 or 18 may not survive long enough to become part of the patient population in a congenital heart clinic. A reasonable estimate would be that 8–10% of congenital heart disease is caused by chromosomal anomalies.

With the increasing recognition that mendelian syndromes have structural and functional cardiovascular abnormalities, and the appreciation that a number of common nonsyndromic, congenital heart lesions may be produced by single mutant genes, we have had to raise our estimate to suggest that 3–5% of congenital heart defects are caused by single genes.

The last line of Table 4-1 will require the most explanation both in this chapter and in the next. New variables are emerging. Suffice it to say that this major category, multifactorial inheritance, to which we presently assign 85% of familial congenital heart cases should be subdivided in the future.

Table 4-1   Etiologic categories of congenital heart diseases

Category	Percentage
Chromosomal anomalies	8–10
Single mutant genes	3–5
Multifactorial inheritance (encompassing environmental interactions)	85

GENERAL OBSERVATIONS

To illustrate some of the difficulties in discovering causes of CHD we may start with some rather simple questions. First, how common is congenital heart disease in defined populations? Among spontaneous abortuses and stillborn fetuses, the prevalence is 13.0% (Chinn et al., 1989). However, Table 4-2 reveals an astonishing range of clinically diagnosed CHD, even allowing for differences in populations, diagnostic criteria, and time frames. In European and North American populations sampled from 1941–1982, the range was 2.08 to 11.7 cases per 1000 (Nora and Nora, 1988). When we began our studies in the 1960s we used population data from that time period in the United States. The California-Kaiser data (Yerushalmy, 1970) showed 11.7 cases per 1000 and the Collaborative National Institutes of Health study (Mitchell et al., 1971) found 7.67 cases per 1000. We combined the data and used 1% as an admittedly rough

Table 4-2   Frequency rates of congenital heart diseases in defined populations*

Population	Cases/1000	Time frame
Sweden, Gothenburg[a]	6.35	1941–1950
USA, NIH Collaborative[b]	7.67	1956–1965
USA, California-Kaiser[c]	11.7	1960–1966
Denmark[d]	6.14	1963–1973
USA, New England[e]	2.08	1969–1974
USA, Baltimore-Washington[f]	3.70	1981–1982
EUROCAT[g]	1.89-10.75	1979–1982
European Collaborative[g]	6.04±2.53	1986
Switzerland[g]	4.01	1986
Japan[g]	10.6	1985

* Adapted from Nora and Nora (1988).
[a] Carlgren, 1959.
[b] Mitchell, 1971.
[c] Yerushalmy, 1970.
[d] Laursen, 1980.
[e] Fyler, 1980.
[f] Ferencz, 1985.
[g] Pexieder, 1988.

population figure. Two studies in the United States from the 1970s and 1980s have found frequencies of 2.08 (Fyler, 1980) and 3.80 (Ferencz et al., 1985) cases per 1000. Could there have been a 4- to 6-fold greater frequency rate of CHD in the United States in the 1960s than in subsequent decades? If it is real, what could have accounted for this difference? Environmental influences? Teratogens?

But what about the Scandinavian data? There was essentially no change when comparing the time frames 1941–1950 (Carlgren, 1959) with 1963–1973 (Laursen, 1980). The frequency rate remained within a narrow range of 6 cases per 1000. Is the problem, then, more restricted to the United States, whether it be case finding, environmental triggers, or some other explanation? Not if you look at the 1979–1982 European Registry of Congenital Anomalies and Twins (EUROCAT) study (Weatherall, 1983), involving several other European countries. There was a range of 1.89 to 10.75 congenital heart cases per 1000. This wide divergence of results prompted a 1986 European collaborative study (Pexieder, 1988) in which, under stricter guidelines, a range of 5.0 to 10.5 (with a mean of 6.04) was found.

Curiously, at the very time when CHD in general appeared to be decreasing in the United States (in the 1980s), at least one heart lesion, ventricular septal defect (VSD), was reported to be increasing (Oakley et al., 1983). Why? In both the United States and EUROCAT studies there were large differences between centers in what should be reported as a VSD. The "epidemic" of VSD in the United States (Spooner et al., 1988) and the greater frequency of CHD in one European country as compared to another (Pexieder, 1988) could be attributed in part to the criteria used to diagnose VSD. At different centers there is substantial disagreement between protocols as to which patients should be accepted as having congenital heart disease. Requiring confirmatory studies such as heart catheterization, echocardiography, and autopsy will eliminate smaller lesions that are not so likely to attract aggressive investigation. But is a small VSD that may close spontaneously of less genetic-epidemiologic importance than a large VSD? Rubella immunization is another factor that may relate to differences in incidence of CHD in different countries. (Note the last two lines of Table 4-2.) A virologist has told us that rubella is more prevalent in Japan than in many other industrialized nations.

Population frequency rates are of more than academic interest. They are critical in undertaking calculations of heritability. Whatever the problems in determining population frequency rates for congenital heart defects, the best approximation must be used for this purpose. We now suggest a figure in the middle of the range: 6 cases per 1000. At the same time, we emphasize that one should not dismiss differences in frequency rates found in apparently conflicting studies without carefully seeking an explanation.

It has been put forward that the genetic basis for most familial congenital heart diseases is best explained by multifactorial inheritance (Nora, 1968a). In that proposal, and in subsequent proposals, we have reported empiric risk data that we use in counseling. But it should be clearly understood that there are investigators who disagree with certain findings, and who base their disagreement on data bases of comparable size and which were obtained with equally meticulous care. From our own experience we recognize that there are biases inherent in series limited in size to the capacity of one investigative group. One or two large families, which are not representative of the rest of the series, may weight and distort numerators. This is particularly true if heart lesions (and syndromes) caused by single mutant genes are present in the data (e.g., atrial septal defect, atrioventricular canal, pulmonary stenosis, and conotruncal syndromes). Some of the problems in estimating incidence (let alone recurrence risk figures) for only one heart lesion, VSD, have been mentioned and will be developed further. Although far from ideal, we feel that combining data from studies of comparable design provides more reliable answers than single studies of inadequate size.

What we would like to do is present principles of recurrence risk counseling which are not locked into precise numbers carried to two decimal places. We will provide the numbers, however, and will combine the data from as many relevant series as we are familiar with into a consensus number and acknowledge the sources of the combined data. We will also suggest a recurrence risk rounded to the nearest 0.5%. Our hope is that this will be a reasonable basis for counseling.

Some definitions are in order. When we use the term multifactorial inheritance in this presentation, we mean a specific mode of inheritance in which *genetic predisposition is presumed to interact with an environmental trigger to produce the trait or abnormality of interest*. The genetic predisposition is most often assumed to be polygenic, but this is not a necessary requirement of multifactorial inheritance, as the term is used here. One or several environmental agents may thus be visualized as interacting with only a single gene.

We have found, as a not invariable rule, that the more common the cardiovascular lesion, the more likely it, or a functionally or structurally related lesion is likely to recur in first-degree relatives. This is consistent with and is predicted by various models of multifactorial inheritance. The risk of VSD recurring in a family should be much greater than the risk of tricuspid atresia. It must be emphasized here that Anderson (1976), in a series comparable in size to ours, does not find that the more common the heart lesion the more likely it is to recur.

A general concept in multifactorial inheritance is that if two first-degree relatives are affected, the recurrence risk for the next child becomes two to three times as great (Table 4-3). If there are three affected first-degree relatives, the recurrence risk is greatly increased. We have called such families type C families (Fig. 4-1), and counsel that the recurrence risk is likely to be that which has already been experienced in the family, whether the etiology is multifactorial, dominant, or even mitochondrial inheritance.

Table 4-3 Recurrence risks (%) for multifactorial diseases according to number of affected first-degree relatives and heritability*

Population frequency (%)	Affected parents Heritability (%)	0 Affected sibs			1 Affected Sibs			2 Affected sibs		
		0	1	2	0	1	2	0	1	2
1.0	100	1	7	14	11	24	34	63	65	67
	80	1	6	14	8	18	28	41	47	52
	50	1	4	8	4	9	15	15	21	26
0.1	100	0.1	4	11	5	16	26	62	63	64
	80	0.1	3	10	4	14	23	60	61	62
	50	0.1	1	3	1	3	7	7	11	15

* Adapted from Smith (1971).

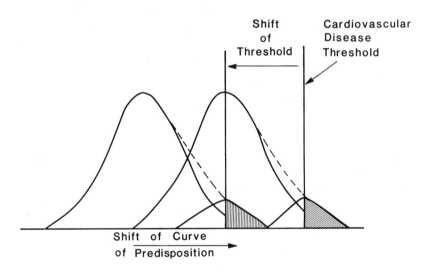

Figure 4-1 Hypothetical quasi-continuous and discontinuous models for multifactorial inheritance of congenital heart diseases. In the typical low-risk (type B) family, the threshold of malformation may be crossed by a symmetrical curve of polygenic predisposition or by a slightly skewed curve in which there is a population with mendelian risks (shaded area). In the type C high-risk family, the normally distributed curve of predisposition moves to the right, and the threshold to the left, accounting for all of the risk in the quasi-continuous models of Falconer and Edwards. Only in the presence of significant dominance may Morton's model be appreciated as accounting for a small portion of families at risk. Although the overall empiric recurrence risk figures are the same in all three models, the risks in a given family must be specifically identified as high- or low-risk on the basis of the individual pedigree.

Such counseling goes beyond theoretic recurrence risks for multifactorial inheritance, such as those of Smith (Table 4-3). Please note that in high heritability, if the two affected first-degree relatives are a parent and a sib, the risk is higher than for two affected sibs. To counsel a high recurrence risk if there are no affected parents is not consistent with the usual expectation in multifactorial inheritance, if one can assume that one or both parents do not have a forme fruste of the malformation. This assumption is difficult to make for lesions such as VSD, for which there is evidence that 30–70% close spontaneously. It is quite possible that there has been a spontaneous closure in presumably normal parents of affected children in type C families. And we have some historical evidence of "disappearing murmurs" in such parents.

Our position regarding high-risk type C families is to utilize empiric risk data when they exist and theoretic risk data when empiric data are not available. *We consider the experience within an individual family to represent the basis for counseling* (Nora and Nora, 1978a) and would certainly not counsel anything but a high risk for the family in Figure 4-2, despite the fact that neither parent had evidence of VSD in adult life. We now suspect that one or both parents had spontaneously closing defects in infancy or that the mother may have had a spontaneously closing defect (this family could possibly represent mitochondrial inheritance, which will be discussed later).

PATHOGENESIS

A difficult question that arises in the analysis of families is: what is the underlying mechanism of maldevelopment in a given family? If VSD appears to be the anomaly running in the family, is the sib recurrence risk of 3% the risk for VSD (see Table 4-4)? Must the population risks for other congenital heart diseases, such as atrial septal defect and patent ductus arteriosus be added to the empiric risk figure?

There are several closely related views of pathogenesis. If one perceives differences in the views, we believe that these are more a matter of emphasis rather than differences of basic concepts. We feel that under the assumption of multifactorial inheritance in a given family, there is an

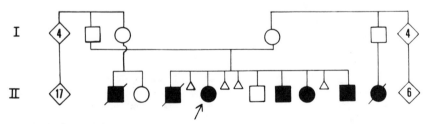

Figure 4-2   High-risk (type C) family with ventricular septal defect (see text).

Table 4-4 Recurrence risks in sibs for any congenital heart defect: combined data published during two decades from European and North American populations. Suggested risk rounded to nearest 0.5%

Defect	1968–1990 Risk (%)	Suggested Risk (%)	
		if 1 sib affected	if 2 sibs affected
Ventricular septal defect	3.2[a–d,i,k]	3	10
Hypoplastic left heart	3.2[a,d,j,m]	3	10
Patent ductus	3.1[a–e,g,k]	3	10
Atrial septal defect	2.7[a–g,k]	2.5	8
Endocardial cushion	2.5[a–d]	2.5	10
Tetralogy of Fallot	2.4[a–d,k]	2.5	8
Pulmonary stenosis	2.2[a–d,k]	2	6
Coarctation of aorta	2.1[a–e]	2	6
Aortic stenosis	2.0[a–d,h]	2	6
Transposition	1.4[a–d,i]	1.5	5
Truncus*	4.1[a,d,l]	1–4	3–12
Pulmonary atresia*	1.2[a,d]	1	3
Tricuspid atresia*	1.0[a,i]	1	3
Ebstein anomaly*	0.9[a,d]	1	3
Interrupted aortic arch*	2.0[d,l]	1–2	3–6

[a] Nora (1968, 1978, 1983, 1988).
[b] Anderson (1976).
[c] Sanchez-Cascos (1978).
[d] Boughman et al. (1987).
[e] Zetterquist, (1972).
[f] Williamson (1969).
[g] Jorgenson and Buren (1971).
[h] Zoethout et al. (1964).
[i] Fuhrmann (1968, 1969).
[j] Holmes et al. (1972).
[k] Mori (1973).
[l] Pierpont (1988).
[m] Morris (1990).
* Provisional.

interaction between a genetic predisposition (usually the product of many genes, but perhaps as few as one gene) and an environmental trigger (e.g., drug, virus, maternal nutrition, or fetal hemodynamics). If the interaction between abnormalities of the very same primary gene products (structural proteins or enzymes) and the same environmental trigger occur at one gestational age, a VSD may result. If the insult is a few days earlier, tetralogy of Fallot may occur, or if a few dates later, atrial septal defect may be produced—all on the basis of the same genetic predisposition and environmental interaction.

Continuing with the example of VSD, human studies and animal experiments reveal that a specific abnormality tends to run in families. In 30–60% of affected sibs of patients with VSD, the lesion is also VSD (Nora and

Nora, 1978b). But this means that 40–70% of the sibs have another heart lesion. This is similar to what we found in the C57BL/6J mouse (Nora et al., 1968b) with teratogenic exposure to amphetamine on day 8 of gestation (61% VSD; 39% other heart lesions). The closure of the ventricular septum is a critically timed event requiring the simultaneous arrival of contributions from the endocardial cushions, the conus, and the interventricular septum. About 50% of all patients who have congenital cardiovascular lesions have VSDs alone (25%) or in combination with other anomalies of the heart (25%). But as common as VSD is, it is a wonder that 99.7% of older infants do not have persistence of this anomaly because of the critical timing required for the completion of the embryologic event. There does appear to be a mechanism to compensate for the failure of the ventricular septum to close at 44 days conceptional age, which is reflected by the large number of cases of late spontaneous closure.

One cannot be sure in a single case what the core lesion that is "running in the family" really is. The first child may have VSD, the second may have tetralogy of Fallot. We would counsel the worst case scenario for the heart lesion (i.e., tetralogy), and would in this family regard VSD as a forme fruste of the complete tetralogy. Parents want to know what the chance is that their next child will have a congenital heart lesion, and are not as interested in the pros and cons regarding predisposition to, versus protection from heart lesions other than the one present in the proband.

We assume that the heart lesions in the first-degree relatives are more likely to be related to the same developmental abnormalities rather than to different ones. Clusters of similar anomalies in families appear to support this (Fraser and Hunter, 1975). A familial recurrence of a heart lesion that apparently bears no developmental relationship to a previously encountered defect may indeed be unrelated (or may be a manifestation of a common mechanism of maldevelopment that is obscure to the observer).

Clark (1986) has developed a construct of cardiac malformation related to right and left heart blood flow and mesenchymal cell migration among other factors. He suggests a classification based on a developmental-mechanistic approach consisting of five basic groups:

   I. abnormal cell migration;
   II. flow lesions;
   III. cell death;
   IV. extracellular matrix;
   V. targeted growth defects.

It is easy to visualize these events taking place within a cascade that would begin with a genetic-environmental interaction. This will be discussed in greater detail in the next chapter.

The neural crest appears to play a critical role in the development of the heart and great vessels. Injury to the neural crest may be important in the production of multiple malformation syndromes (McCredie, 1976) as well as in cardiovascular maldevelopment. The postganglionic neurons innervating the heart are derived from the neural crest and the ectomesenchyme required for septation of the outflow tract and proper development of the aortic arch arteries come from the same level of the neural crest as the parasympathetic postganglionic innervation (Kirby, 1987, 1988). Removal of the cardiac area of the neural crest causes structural and functional changes commensurate with the amount of tissue removed. Malformation syndromes to be defined later, such as the CHARGE (coloboma of the eye, heart anomaly, atresia, retardation, genital, and ear abnormalities), conotruncal anomaly face (Shimizu et al., 1984), DiGeorge, Goldenhar, velocardiofacial, and possibly VACTERL (vertebral, anal, cardiac, tracheaesophageal, renal, limb) syndromes may illustrate this mechanism. Also, a number of drugs that produce malformation syndromes, including thalidomide, retinoic acid, alcohol, and possibly hydantoin and exogenous sex hormones could be visualized as having the potential to injure the neural crest through various means (e.g., reactive intermediates). Certainly, in experimental animals, drugs such as bis-diamine produce conotruncal anomalies (Okamoto et al., 1984) and thymic aplasia, cryptorchism, facial and other anomalies (Ikeda et al., 1984).

As we have stated earlier in this section, we feel that the essential factors in the multifactorial inheritance of congenital cardiovascular defects are a genetic predisposition to a form of maldevelopment, which can be triggered by one or several possible environmental influences (to which there is also a genetic predisposition), and that the exact form of the maldevelopment will depend on the embryologic timing of the environmental insult. It is also clear that certain environmental agents produce characteristic anomalies (as we will explore later).

For defects produced by multifactorial inheritance, there appears to be a higher risk of disease to offspring of affected parents than to sibs of patients. At least for CHD, however, the risk to offspring of affected mothers exceeds expectation as compared to offspring of affected fathers or affected sibs. In general, the recurrence risk in sibs as shown in Table 4-4 is in the range of 1–3% with a higher risk being found for the more common lesions (e.g., VSD versus tricuspid atresia). The matrilineal risk (as opposed to patrilineal and sib risks) will be scrutinized in later sections.

GENETIC MODES AND MODELS

In a search for a suitable genetic explanation of familial recurrence of congenital heart diseases, we were able to reject single-gene and chromosomal etiologies in the *majority* of cases (Nora, 1968a). However, these two genetic modes account for conceptually and clinically important subgroups, which are best handled in separate chapters. On the basis of our early data and our continuing experience, we are not able to reject multifactorial inheritance as the etiologic explanation for most familial cases of

CHD. Three models of multifactorial inheritance frequently referred to in the literature are those of Falconer, Edwards, and Morton.

According to Falconer's (Falconer, 1965) model, liability to a disease represents the total of genetic and environmental influences. The heritability of liability may be estimated from a continuous normally distributed variable. Edwards' (Edwards, 1969) model assumes that the probability of being affected increases exponentially as the liability increases. Discontinuity is introduced in Morton's (Morton et al., 1970) model with the concept that a disease may be determined by rare single genes in a small number of cases and the small effects of many genes in most cases.

All three models fit the data for most congenital heart diseases. We currently find Morton's model to be more appealing and better able to explain the family studies (e.g., atrial septal defect) than the alternative models. However, in any model of multifactorial inheritance, we consider the contribution of the environment to be of major importance.

In light of newly recognized modes of inheritance, it may be necessary to reexamine many common disorders presently considered to be best explained as multifactorial. Three other possibilities should at least be tentatively mentioned here: mitochondrial inheritance, genomic imprinting, and germline mosaicism.

Some of us have for many years quoted recurrence risk figures in CHD for first-degree relatives on the assumption that although the risk to a child of an affected parent is usually higher than to a sib of a proband—as shown in Table 4-3 of Smith (1971)—the risks are only moderately higher. In preparing this updated volume, we reviewed the parent-offspring risks in our own series and in other published series that provided specific information on risks to offspring of affected parents (Table 4-5). We were astonished to find that the risks to offspring are much higher from affected

Table 4-5 Suggested offspring recurrence risk for congenital heart defects given 1 affected parent based on combined data* and rounded to the nearest 0.5%

Defect	Mother affected	Father affected
Aortic stenosis	18	5
Atrial septal defect	6	1.5
Coarctation of aorta	4	2.5
Endocardial cushion defect	14**	1
Patent ductus arteriosus	4	2
Pulmonary stenosis	6.5	2
Tetralogy of Fallot	2.5	1.5
Ventricular septal defect	9.5	2.5

* Nora (1969, 1978, 1983, 1987, 1988); Williamson (1969); Taussig (1971); Zetterqvist (1972); Dennis (1981); Whittemore (1982); Czeizel (1982); Emanuel et al. (1983); Rose (1985); Ferencz (1986).
** Provisional.

mothers than the risks from affected fathers. Most of the series were small, and in one instance, where the authors (Czeizel et al., 1982) analyzed the differences in risk related to the sex of the affected parent, the numbers did not reach statistical significance. Other groups, including our own, did not even attempt an analysis for the sex of the affected parent until recently.

What is difficult to deny is that in series after series, whether specifically analyzed by the authors or not, the high risk is from the mother rather than the father (Nora and Meyer, 1966; Taussig et al., 1971; Zetterquist, 1972; Dennis and Warren, 1981; Czeizel et al., 1982; Emanuel et al., 1983). In a study confined to offspring of affected mothers, Whittemore et al. (1982) found substantially higher recurrence risks than previous investigators. Ferencz (1986), in a study limited to affected fathers, reported unusually low offspring recurrence risks. Rose et al. (1985) found that for three lesions the recurrence risk is higher if the mother is affected, but that the risk from affected fathers is also higher than in many series. In data unpublished at the time of this writing, Whittemore suggests that the risk to offspring of affected males with congenital heart disease is almost as high as in females if one eliminates various cases, including those in which there is a strong family history. But of course, the cases with a strong family history are the very ones that are of genetic interest. We should emphasize that the recurrence risk data we use in counseling combines all the series we can find—high-risk and low-risk.

There are several possible explanations for the finding of higher risk from affected mothers, including maternal vulnerability to teratogens (which will be discussed in the next chapter). Another explanation that deserves mention here is mitochondrial (or cytoplasmic) inheritance. The crucial function of mitochondrial enzymes in energy transformation does nothing to reduce suspicion of these organelles as they may participate in normal and abnormal structural development (although only a few diseases are attributed to this recently recognized mode of inheritance at the present time). We and others have a number of families in which *matrilineal transmission of CHD occurs in almost all offspring*. Some of these are three-generation families (see Fig. 4-3). Although there may not be many such families, only a few are needed to influence (or skew) overall recurrence risk data. In counseling families in which there is an affected mother, the higher recurrence risk than for the child of an affected father must be revealed. But how high is the risk after one affected child? How high is the risk after two affected children? When does the possibility of mitochondrial inheritance become less than remote? Certainly one would require that the transmission of the defect be greater than for dominant inheritance.

And what of the possibility of genomic imprinting (Swain et al., 1988; Hall and Edwards, 1989)? When a disorder does not follow the expectations for regular mendelian inheritance, other explanations must be explored. Differential expression of maternal genetic information *exclusively* might be considered in the above data, but one would prefer that there be

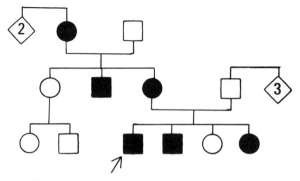

Figure 4-3 Three-generation high-risk family with atrial septal defect.

comparable evidence of differential expression of paternal genetic contribution in some families or for some lesions. The parental origin of the deletion of chromosome 15 in Angelman syndrome is almost entirely maternal, and in Prader-Willi syndrome it is almost entirely paternal (Knoll et al., 1989). We are not presently familiar with a clear-cut paternal contribution in congenital heart defects. At this very early stage of investigation of imprinting, we feel that this may ultimately prove to be an important etiologic consideration in common disorders, including CHD.

In familial disorders restricted to sibs, germline mosaicism is a recently emphasized potential mode of inheritance (Edwards, 1989). However, most congenital heart diseases compatible with survival to the age of reproduction show evidence of direct transmission. We must continue to stress that counseling should be based on the specific experience within the family.

Although Table 4-5 is our most recent revision and incorporates information not present in our previous publications, we feel that considerably more smoothing of these data will take place over the next few years. There are certainly too few familial cases of endocardial cushion defect to accept a 14% recurrence risk for offspring of affected mothers. Even a small number of high-risk families can skew the data. The high risk may come from dominant or even mitochondrial inheritance. The unusually high risk for children of mothers with aortic stenosis is present in three series now. This will be discussed in the section on that defect.

Genetic counselors will want to use specific risk figures as shown in Table 4-5 with the reservation that the exact numbers are subject to change as new data become available. In general, the *risk of transmitting a congenital heart disease appears to be two to five times greater if the affected parent is the mother.*

In the section that follows, a brief review of empiric and theoretic risks for various congenital heart lesions will be offered. Where applicable, teratogenic, epidemiologic, and genetic relationships of special importance in a given lesion will be discussed. Those instances of substantial disagreement in the literature will also be noted.

SPECIFIC ANOMALIES

Differences in recurrence risks are evident when comparing various series in the literature. Fuhrmann's (Fuhrmann, 1968; Fuhrmann and Vogel, 1969) cases are restricted to recurrence of the same or of a related abnormality. Anderson's (1976) series admits patients who do not have concordant cardiac anomalies, but eliminates patients having syndromes of known or unknown etiology and a variety of teratogenic exposures, including diabetes and anticonvulsants, which have been implicated in cardiovascular maldevelopment. Zetterquist (1972) reports familial recurrence of concordant and discordant lesions and emphasizes that it is the concordant lesions that are of greater genetic interest. We have reported familial recurrence of congenital cardiovascular disease whether they are concordant or are apparently discordant types because we felt that the basic mechanisms of maldevelopment were not yet clearly defined. We felt also that the meaningful figure in counseling is the recurrence of a congenital cardiovascular defect, not the recurrence of a specific lesion per se. In the past we eliminated only chromosomal and single-gene etiologies and rubella. We have previously stated:

> There is much to be learned from analysis of concordant and discordant cardiovascular anomalies within families. It may turn out that we should not group anomalies by pathologic diagnosis, e.g. tetralogy of Fallot or ventricular septal defect, but rather by pathogenesis, e.g., abnormalities of truncoconal septation or endocardial cushion formation. We would, of course, have to revise our theoretic recurrence risks, which are based on traditional diagnoses, imprecise formulas and uncertain population frequencies (Nora and Nora, 1978b).

Clark (1986) and others are currently following this investigative direction.

For our empiric risk records, we do not eliminate recurrence associated with syndromes of unknown etiology, or potential teratogens which are not established as high-risk (and may or may not have played an etiologic role). Eventually, as more teratogens are identified, the recurrences attributable to these agents may bring the nonteratogen-related recurrences to a much lower level. The genetic-environmental interaction continues to be the focus of our interest. We forcefully stress the need to avoid unnecessary exposures to drugs and other potential environmental hazards in the pregnancies that will follow the delivery of an infant with congenital cardiovascular disease.

Finally, it will be observed that as increasing numbers of cases are published, it is both reasonable and necessary to combine data to reduce the discrepancies produced by outlying observations in individual series. It has been somewhat painful to modify the empiric counseling figures we have used over the years that have been derived from our own research. But this is all related to the increasing knowledge of the subject. It is likely that high-risk families having single-gene etiologies have previously been mixed in with families having presumed multifactorial inheritance (e.g., dominant atrial septal defect and dominant pulmonary stenosis in unrecognized Noonan syndrome). The value of empiric recurrence risk data is diminishing because the trend is toward greater specificity in etiologic understanding, pathogenesis, and genetic-environmental counseling.

Currently, because most data are based on pathologic diagnoses rather than on conceptual grouping related to tentative assignments of pathogenesis, we will continue to follow this standard (if not entirely satisfactory) convention. In many of the lesions that follow, we could ask the question: could mitochondrial inheritance, genomic imprinting, or germline mosaicism be playing an etiologic role? For conciseness, we will not raise the question for each defect.

Ventricular Septal Defect (VSD)

This most common of congenital heart defects, Ventricular Septal Defect (VSD), is present as an isolated lesion in 0.25% of older infants and children, and in almost an equal number of cases as part of a complex of heart anomalies (e.g., tetralogy of Fallot). The murmur of VSD has been found in about 3% of a subsample taken from 2000 newborns evaluated as controls in a study of potential teratogenic agents in congenital cardiovascular disease (Nora et al., 1978c). In the past, enough patients with similar murmurs have had documentation by cardiac catheterization of small VSDs to make catheterization of such infants clinically unjustified and meddlesome. This apparently high frequency of spontaneously closing VSDs has important implications in genetic counseling. Where should the threshold for diagnosing a VSD be set?

One approach has been to disregard these murmurs and to not record the infants as having significant VSDs if the murmur disappeared within three months (and if there was no other evidence of cardiovascular disease). While this approach prevents overestimating the occurrence of significant heart disease in teratogenic studies, it may obscure another issue. Physicians for many decades have disregarded "disappearing murmurs" and indeed, until recently, did not appreciate those that represented small, spontaneously closing, VSDs. We are becoming more convinced that from the genetic point of view, a VSD that closes spontaneously at three days of age has implications of hereditary predisposition. As discussed in the introduction to this chapter, in the high-risk type C families in which recurrence in sibs greatly exceeds expectation for multifactorial inheritance, it is possible that one or both parents had spontaneously closing VSDs.

The recurrence risks that we now give are shown in Table 4-4. This figure is based on the small series of Boughman et al. (1987), which yields the highest recurrence risk (5.8%), and our series (4.3%) combined with four other series that have lower recurrence risks. The sib recurrence risk from the combined data of six series is 3.2%, which we round to 3%. If there are two affected sibs, we counsel an increase in risk three times greater than for one affected sib (i.e., about 10%). If there are three affected first-degree relatives, we counsel that the risk will be high, possibly as high as has already been experienced in the family. Our recurrence risk in sibs is higher than that found by Anderson (1976), Furhmann (1969), Mori (1973), or Sanchez-Cascos (1978), and may be related to differing methods of case selection (as described in the previous section and in the introduction to this section) and to the presence in our series of some rather striking type C families.

The recurrence risk that we counsel for the presence of cardiovascular disease in an offspring, given one parent with a VSD, is 9.5% if the mother is affected and 1.5% if the father has VSD, based on six series of cases. The frequency of concordant heart lesions recurring in first-degree relatives of a proband presenting with VSD varies from 30–60% depending on the series. Tetralogy of Fallot is the most common discordant lesion in our experience and in that of Fraser and Hunter (1975). But in these families, we are inclined to consider tetralogy of Fallot to be the lesion of concern (representing a more profound predisposition) and VSD to be the forme fruste of tetralogy. Ostium secundum atrial septal defect is next most common, followed by transposition of the great arteries, pulmonary valve stenosis, patent ductus arteriosus, aortic stenosis, coarctation of the aorta, truncus arteriosus, tricuspid atresia, and dextroversion.

Ventricular septal defect is the most common cardiac malformation associated with a number of teratogenic insults, including alcohol, progestogen/estrogen, amphetamines, anticonvulsants, and retinoic acid. Since it is also the most common congenital heart defect, no exceptional relationship can be deduced from this information other than that environmental triggers are apparently playing an important interactive role.

Males and females are affected with approximately equal frequency, and no striking epidemiologic finding regarding birth order, parental age, season of birth, area of residence, ethnic origin, or socioeconomic level has emerged.

Hypoplastic Left Heart Syndrome (HLHS)

In a geographically defined population (Oregon), Hypoplastic Left Heart Syndrome (HLHS) occurred in 0.162 per 1000 live births (Morris et al., 1990). HLHS represents about 8% of congenital heart disease and has the second highest sib recurrence risk (3.2%) as determined from combined data of six series of cases from 9 locations (Holmes et al., 1972; Boughman et al., 1987; Morris et al., 1990). This recurrence risk is higher than one would predict for multifactorial inheritance alone (based on the population frequency of HLHS). Only about 25% of recurrences are HLHS, the remaining cases include a variety of anomalies: aortic anomalies, ventricular and atrial septal defects, truncus, and left-sided outflow lesions. Because HLHS has been incompatible with survival to the reproductive age, there are no offspring data. Recent surgical advances such as the Norwood procedure should alter this expectation. However, 1.2% of infants with HLHS have a parent with another form of CHD. Congenital brain anomalies have been reported in 29% of 41 infants with HLHS (Glauser et al., 1990). Occasional associations with teratogens have been reported, but none are striking or specific.

There has been one report that is consistent with HLHS being autosomal recessive (Shokeir, 1971). In this study there were 15 individuals with HLHS in 6 families with 9 sibships. In 5 families there was consanguinity. These findings were in the province of Saskatchewan, Canada. One possible explanation for the striking difference between the data from Saskatchewan and the other locations could be that there is a recessive gene more common in this population. However, the finding that 5 of 38 sibs of HLHS patients in the Baltimore-Washington Infant Study (Ferencz et al., 1985) had congenital heart disease could suggest a recessive gene in some families. The fact that the sib recurrence risk of HLHS appears to be greater than the expectation for multifactorial inheritance may thus reflect a mendelian mix (or the possibility of one of the more recently described modes such as mitochondrial inheritance or imprinting).

We counsel a 3% risk for some form of CHD after one child with a hypoplastic left heart. After two affected infants, we feel that autosomal recessive inheritance should also be considered.

Patent Ductus Arteriosus (PDA)

Patent Ductus Arteriosus (PDA) is in many series the second most common congenital cardiovascular anomaly, accounting for about 10% of congenital heart defects. Females are more often affected (M : F 1 : 2) except in rubella-related disease. In our own series, to date, 3.2% of sibs of probands with PDA have a congenital heart lesion. Zetterquist found 2.5% of sibs to have a congenital cardiovascular anomaly. Jorgensen and Beuren (1971) reported 3.7% of sibs to be affected. Anderson found no significant increase in congenital heart lesions in sibs over the population frequency. The combined sib recurrence risk from six series is 3.1%. The risk to offspring of mothers with PDA, based on four series is 4.1%, and the risk to offspring of affected fathers is 2.2%.

Concordance is somewhat variable between series. This is probably related to the reporting of isolated PDA versus PDA associated with other defects. If a proband has PDA alone, the chance that the cardiovascular anomaly in a first-degree relative will also be PDA alone is greater than 50%. If PDA is associated with other defects, the chance of isolated PDA being present in a first-degree relative is much less than 50%. Anomalies associated with PDA or found (with or without PDA) in first-degree relatives of probands with PDA (with or without associated anomalies) include the following in approximate descending order of frequency: VSD, coarctation of the aorta, transposition of the great arteries, tetralogy of Fallot, atrial septal defect, endocardial cushion defect, aortic stenosis, and tricuspid atresia. It appears that isolated PDA and PDA associated with other cardiac defects represent two different problems.

The teratogenic implications in PDA have received considerable attention. Rubella virus is the most prominent teratogen in the etiology of PDA. The ductus seems most vulnerable during the first trimester, with relatively few examples of suspected teratogenic effect in the second trimester, and no cases of rubella-related patent ductus attributed to third trimester events. This is curious because rubella virus has been shown to be responsible for progression of disease in the pulmonary artery branches even during postnatal life and is present in newborn infants with maternal rubella syndrome. The ductus is also highly vulnerable to fluid overload in premature newborns. It is reasonable to believe that although various teratogenic influences in the etiology of PDA are mainly first-trimester events, the ductus may remain vulnerable throughout pregnancy.

Season of birth, birth rank, and parental age have not been implicated, but high altitude residence has been proposed as a possible etiologic factor in one study.

Atrial Septal Defect (ASD)

The frequency of atrial septal defect (ASD) approximates 10% of congenital heart disease and is found predominantly in females (M : F 1 : 2). The recurrence risks of a congenital cardiac anomaly if there is one affected sib is 2.9% in our series, 3.7% in the series of Williamson (1969), 4.6% in the series of Jorgensen and Beuren, and about 1% or less in studies by Anderson and of Zetterquist. The figure we use for recurrence in the next sib of a patient with ASD is 2.5%, which is rounded from 2.7% found by combining seven studies. For the offspring of mothers with ASD, the risk is 6.2% found by combining five studies, and the risk from affected fathers is 1.7% found by combining five studies (Nora and Nora, 1987).

There are examples (in our series and in the series of others) of direct transmission of ASD through three generations. ASD is found in several mendelian syndromes, including the dominant ASD with prolonged P-R interval, Holt-Oram and Noonan syndromes, and the recessive Ellis-van Creveld and thrombocytopenia-absent-radius syndromes. It is likely that every series that has an intake of high-risk families has cases of true mendelian transmission, which are masquerading as multifactorial inheritance and "padding" the empiric recurrence risk figures. Our series could have such a bias. We look carefully for evidence of slight fingerization of the thumb or other forme fruste of a dominant syndrome. Even without other stigmata we counsel a high recurrence risk of 50%, not 6%, in a family such as that shown in Figure 4-4.

Our experience with ASD has influenced our thinking regarding models of multifactorial inheritance. At least for ASD, Morton's model seems most compatible with what we have found in our series. While polygenes

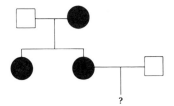

Figure 4-4   Potentially high-risk family with atrial septal defect. The empiric risk for the first child should not be based on the premise of only one affected first-degree relative when the possibility of dominant inheritance is strongly suggested by the pedigree.

may underlie many familial cases, rare single genes appear to have an etiologic role in other families with ASD.

However, an autosomal dominant bias should affect matrilineal and patrilineal inheritance equally. Why then is maternal transmission of ASD four times higher than paternal? By conventional expectation in multifactorial inheritance, because females are affected more often than males, it is assumed that a greater genetic burden is required to produce the lesion in the male and this greater burden translates to a higher recurrence risk to offspring of affected males. However, this is not what is found in ASD (and to a lesser extent in PDA). The higher recurrence risk is to the offspring of females. Maternal vulnerability to teratogens? Mitochondrial inheritance? Imprinting?

Concordance in sibs and first-degree relatives of patients with ASD is about 50% in combined series. (Concordance of heart malformation in A/J mice treated with amphetamines is 67%). The most common discordant lesion in humans is VSD, followed by pulmonary stenosis, aortic stenosis, transposition of the great arteries, and tricuspid atresia.

ASD is frequently found in offspring whose mothers have had various teratogenic exposures. There has been no highly characteristic relationship, however, such as is found between rubella virus in PDA, and lithium in Ebstein anomaly. Some seasonal variation in birth has been reported, but there are enough differences between series to diminish the value of this observation. Birth order, parental age, area of residence, and ethnic origin have not been identified as playing a significant etiologic role.

Endocardial Cushion Defect (ECD)

In our first 70 families ascertained through a proband who had an endocardial cushion defect (ECD), we found no recurrence in sibs. Then we found one striking family (Fig. 4-5) that changed our empiric risk data from 0% to 2.6% (4/151). Anderson found a recurrence in sibs of probands with ECD of 1.5% (2/132), and Emanuel et al. (1968) a recurrence risk of 1.8% in first-degree relatives in the initial report of their series. Sanchez-Cascos (1978) reported a frequency of 8.7% (14/161) of congenital heart diseases among first-degree relatives of probands with ECD. These data illustrate the problem introduced by possible outliers in relatively small series. The sib recurrence risk based on four series is 2.5%. A major concern in ECD is that when it is familial, it may be high-risk (type C or mendelian). Emanuel

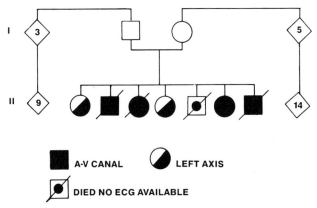

A-V CANAL

LEFT AXIS

DIED NO ECG AVAILABLE

Figure 4-5 Even in relatively uncommon lesions, such as endocardial cushion defect, there can be unusual high-risk families with a mendelian or a polygenic basis. The recurrence risk in this family obviously would not be 2%, but would be based on what has been experienced in the family. The left axis deviation may be regarded as a forme fruste of endocardial cushion defect and may be taken to mean that the offspring of those with left axis deviation are also at risk.

et al. (1983) have the only specific parent-offspring series. They found a risk to offspring of 9.6% in this second report of their series. If it was the mother who had the heart defect, however, the risk to offspring was 14%, and 0% if it was the father. This is based on only 35 mothers and 16 fathers, so these data must be used with reservation, until larger numbers become available. We use a 1% patrilineal recurrence risk to emphasize that a zero risk is incompatible with expectations for the general population.

Concordance in all series is high (≈90%)—higher than for other structural anomalies. Patent ductus arteriosus is the most common discordant anomaly, but there is no spectrum of anomalies as is found in transposition of the great arteries, tetralogy of Fallot, VSD, pulmonary stenosis, and ASD (this is compatible with a common pathogenesis for these lesions with a difference in timing of the environmental influence). Indeed, teratogenic exposures are not reported in ECD. This suggests that environmental factors play a lesser role in ECD and that the pathogenesis is different from the other common heart defects just enumerated. An additional related finding is that left axis deviation (anterior fascicular block), which is considered an important electrocardiographic feature of ECD, has been found by us and by others in family members who do not have evidence of atrioventricular (AV) canal or other structural abnormalities of ECD. We have regarded left axis deviation in these patients as a forme fruste of the more complete disease and feel that their offspring are also at risk.

Males and females are affected equally, and factors such as birth order, parental age and seasonal variation have not been identified as being of etiologic significance.

Tetralogy of Fallot (TOF)

Tetralogy of Fallot (TOF) is a complex malformation that accounts for about 10% of congenital heart defects in North America, but only 3.6% in a European survey from 1979–1982 (Weatherall, 1983). The recurrence risk after one affected sib is 2.9% in our series. In Anderson's series the recurrence in sibs is 1.5%. Combining the data from five series yields a sib recurrence risk of 2.4%. Also on the basis of five series of cases, the recurrence risk for the offspring of a mother with TOF is 2.6%, and 1.5% for the offspring of affected fathers. Although the higher risk is matrilineal, it is less than in any of the other lesions for which there are data, and at this time is no higher for offspring of affected mothers than for recurrence in sibs.

Tetralogy occurs in chromosomal and single-gene syndromes and has been associated with maternal exposure to suspected teratogens, but there is no highly specific association. What appears to be most likely from thalidomide and progestogen/estrogen data on maternal exposures is that tetralogy is associated with very early teratogenic insults. Conotruncal septation is complete by day 34 of fetal development, so it is unlikely that a complete tetralogy could result from an environmental insult later than day 34. However, one could also visualize that in the presence of the same genetic predisposition to cardiac maldevelopment, a later insult would be able to attack only developing structures that are still vulnerable, such as the ventricular septum or the pulmonary outflow tract.

Indeed, pulmonary stenosis and VSD are the two most common "unlike" anomalies found in sibs of patients with tetralogy. Transposition of the great arteries is the next most common, which supports the concept that the basic pathogenetic abnormality in tetralogy is in conotruncal development. Pseudotruncus is the next most common anomaly in sibs, which is not surprising since this anomaly is generally regarded as the most severe form of tetralogy. True tetralogy occurs in less than 50% of sibs of probands with TOF. We suspect that, given 2 sibs with tetralogy, the risk for tetralogy in the next sib would increase 3-fold. However, we only know of 2 examples of 3 sibs with tetralogy.

Males more commonly have TOF than females (M : F 3 : 2). Seasonal variation, birth order, parental age, area of residence, and ethnic origin have not been implicated as significant factors.

Pulmonary Stenosis (PS)

Pulmonary valvular stenosis is approximately as common in U.S. surveys as ASD and TOF—each representing about 10% of CHD. It is found as frequently in males as in females (M : F 1 : 1) and has some striking associations, with both teratogenic exposures and single mutant gene syndromes.

Rubella virus produced pulmonary artery branch stenosis, with or without pulmonary valve stenosis, in 55% of patients in our series in Houston during the 1964–1965 pandemic. Data from this series and from the Collaborative Natural History Study reveal that 2% of patients diagnosed as having pulmonary stenosis (PS) during the 1960s, during and following the pandemic, had rubella syndrome.

In our cardiac clinic population, in the 1970s, about 10% of our patients with PS had Noonan syndrome. Pulmonary stenosis is found in other autosomal dominant syndromes, such as neurofibromatosis and Leopard syndrome, and in the recessive Weill-Marchesani syndrome.

From the point of view of genetic counseling, it is essential to determine the presence or absence of mendelian and teratogenic modes before going into empiric risk figures (which exclude single-gene mutations and rubella). If Noonan syndrome is present in a patient with PS, the risk of Noonan syndrome is 50%, and the risk of some form of cardiovascular disease is about 25% (since approximately half of individuals with Noonan syndrome have cardiovascular involvement). This is an entirely different order of risk from that in multifactorial inheritance, so it is essential that one look carefully for stigmata of Noonan or other syndromes.

In our series, excluding rubella and mendelian disorders, the recurrence risk in sibs is 2.7%. Anderson found 1.5% recurrence in sibs. The combined data of five studies yield a sib recurrence risk of 2.2%. The matrilineal recurrence risk is 6.5% and the patrilineal risk is 2%, each based on the combined data of five studies.

Coarctation of the Aorta (CA)

Coarctation of the aorta (CA) is found more commonly in males (M : F 2 : 1) and represents about 7% of congenital cardiovascular disease. Our family study, among others, does not encompass preductal CA. It is the characteristic cardiovascular lesion in Turner syndrome, and is seen occasionally in some mendelian syndromes. It is not frequently found in suspected teratogenic situations, except in infants of diabetic mothers.

The recurrence risk of some form of cardiovascular disease in sibs of probands having CA is 1.8% in both our series and in Zetterquist's series. In Anderson's series it is 0.6%, and in Jorgensen's series 2%. The combined sib recurrence risk in five series is 2.1%. The occurrence of cardiovascular disease in the offspring of mothers with CA is 4.2%, and for fathers 2.3%. The concordance in sibs of probands having CA is comparable to what is found in most other cardiac defects—about 50%.

Aortic stenosis or a bicuspid aortic valve occurs in over half of patients with CA. It is also the most common "unlike" cardiac defect found in sibs of subjects with CA. Patent ductus arteriosus, ASD, and transposition of the great arteries are other discordant anomalies in sibs.

Aortic Stenosis (AS)

Sufficient family data are available on valvular aortic stenosis (AS) to provide some empiric risk figures. Idiopathic hypertrophic subaortic stenosis and supravalvular AS are autosomal dominant disorders and, for subvalvular aortic stenosis, there are insufficient data for counseling (other than through reliance on theoretical risk figures). Valvular AS is found more commonly in males (M : F 2 : 1). It is not found prominently in syndromes of single-gene or chromosomal etiology, except in Turner syndrome. There is also no striking association with specific teratogens. Birth order, parental age, and seasonal variation do not appear to be significant etiologic factors.

Zoethout et al. (1964) found a recurrence risk in sibs of 4% in their series composed mostly of valvular AS, but not specifically excluding other types. Our series is restricted to valvular stenosis and reveals a recurrence risk of 2.2% in sibs. Anderson found a 0.8% frequency of cardiac anomalies in sibs. Combining data from five series we found a risk of 2% for sibs.

The recurrence risk to offspring of mothers with AS, based on four series having a total of 130 probands is 17.7%. The risk to offspring of 138 affected fathers, also based on four series, is 5%. These are the highest matrilineal and patrilineal risks found in any of the eight defects for which there are substantial parent-offspring data. In contrast with the high recurrence risk in ECD based on only 35 mothers and 5 affected children, the 130 mothers and 23 affected children in AS constitute a series of sufficient size to make it difficult to ignore an unusually high recurrence risk and a highly significant difference in matrilineal compared with patrilineal risk. If this striking difference persists between recurrence risks in offspring of affected mothers, and patrilineal and sib risks, it will be essential to explain why.

Sibs of probands with AS have AS alone or in combination with other defects in about 50% of cases. Lesions which may be found in association with AS or as isolated defects in sibs of probands with AS include VSD, PDA, CA, ASD, PS, TOF, and secondary fibroelastosis.

Transposition of the Great Arteries (TGA)

Transposition of the great arteries (TGA) may be approached in 3 ways: restricted to d-transposition, restricted to l-transposition, or mixing the 2 types. Our family data are restricted to probands with d-transposition. Fuhrmann's data include both types, based on the reasonable premise that since both types may occur in the same family, they represent the same disorder of development. About 5% of congenital heart disease in the population is d-transposition. Males are affected more commonly (M : F 2 : 1). At some centers in the United States a definite seasonal trend has been found, with an excess of cases in the spring. Certain potentially teratogenic exposures, including amphetamines, progestogen/estrogen, trimethadione, and maternal diabetes have been followed by cases of TGA. In no syndrome produced by a single mutant gene or a chromosomal anomaly is TGA the most commonly associated cardiovascular abnormality.

In our series, the recurrence risk for a cardiovascular malformation in the sib of a patient with TGA is 1.7%, in Anderson's series 0%, and in Fuhrmann's series 5%. There are no significant data yet on offspring of adults with TGA, but we may anticipate such data in the future from long-term survivors of surgical correction.

About one-third of recurrences in sibs are concordant for TGA. In the other two-thirds, the majority of cases also are in the category of conotruncal maldevelopment (e.g., TOF, truncus arteriosus). Isolated VSD and PDA are also found frequently. A variety of other simple and complex lesions have been reported in sibs.

Teratogenic influences appear to be particularly strong in TGA. Since conotruncal development is completed so early, one should look for very early exposures at a time when the mother may be uncertain as to whether or not she is pregnant. This was of particular relevance when thalidomide and oral hormonal pregnancy tests were still being given.

Less Common Anomalies

There are data concerning several other lesions, which will be briefly cited, but may not be sufficient as a basis for counseling. These defects are separated in Table 4-4 by a horizontal line from the previously described abnormalities and marked with an asterisk to signify that the authors feel that the risk figures should be considered provisional. All that may be reasonably said is that familial cases have been reported. But for rare cardiovascular anomalies, the sib recurrence risks are still not confidently determined. No offspring data can be offered at this time.

Truncus arteriosus has been studied by us in 43 families having 86 sibs. There was one affected sib (pulmonary valvular stenosis). Fraser and Hunter (1975), reporting discordant lesions, found three sibs of probands with truncus to have pulmonary valvular stenosis. Transposition of the great arteries, tetralogy, pseudotruncus, double outlet right ventricle, VSD, and PDA have also been found, which could point to an underlying abnormality in conotruncal development. A recent Minnesota study (Pierpont et al., 1988) of 106 sibs of 49 probands with truncus arteriosus disclosed 7 patients with a cardiovascular defect (6.6%). Single mutant gene conotruncal syndromes and common environmental triggers acting on the neural crest might be considerations in some cases.

Pulmonary valve atresia with intact ventricular septum has not been reported to recur in sibs in our review of the literature, but we have reported PS occurring in the sib of a patient with pulmonary valve atresia. Hypoplastic right ventricle with tricuspid valve hypoplasia has been found in sibs, suggesting that a predisposition to right heart defects may exist in these families, and that the specific manifestation may relate to the timing of the environmental trigger.

Among 98 sibs of 52 probands with tricuspid atresia we have seen only one recurrence of a congenital heart lesion. The sib had a VSD. Fuhrmann (1968) found only one affected sib (with PDA) among 92 sibs of 33 pro-

bands with tricuspid atresia. Fraser, looking specifically for unlike manifestations among sibs with heart anomalies, found PDA, VSD, TOF, PS,
and AS. We have not been able to find an example in the literature of
concordant recurrence in sibs, but we do know of an example of concordance between first cousins. Based on almost 200 sibs from 85 families in the
combined experience of our group and that of Fuhrmann, it appears that
there is a 1% recurrence risk in sibs for some form of congenital heart
disease.

We are familiar with published and unpublished cases of recurrence of
Ebstein anomaly in sibs who are not a part of a series. Our own experience
is limited to one such family. Ebstein anomaly has been reported in an
uncle and nephew (Donegan et al., 1968), and various discordant anomalies have been reported in families and sibships. A genetic predisposition
to this type of maldevelopment probably exists and may be acted upon by
some highly specific teratogens. Lithium is an example of such a teratogen
and is discussed in Chapter 6. The recurrence risk of CHD in sibs is on the
order of 1%.

In a single study involving 36 index cases with interruption of the aortic
arch (IAA), there were 2 sibs with congenital cardiovascular malformations among 98 (2.1%). IAA is found in about 20% of patients with
DiGeorge syndrome.

PERSPECTIVE ON THE DATA

Although congenital heart disease as a general category is one, if not the
most common, of structural anomalies, the data are deficient if the investi-
gator wishes to look at distinct pathologic or pathogenetic entities. Indeed,
the data may even be deficient in reaching a simple answer as to frequency
rates of CHD in given populations. We noted earlier that the frequency of
CHD in Scandinavia remained around 0.6% during the comparative time
frames 1941–1950 and 1963–1973, yet there was an apparent great variation in EUROCAT in the 1980s, and in the United States between the 1960s
and 1970s. The EUROCAT data were eventually smoothed after subsequent study.

Perhaps it is useful to narrow the focus to one lesion, VSD, over which
there has been considerable discussion regarding recent prevalence rates.
A reported 4-fold increase in VSD comparing 1970 to 1983 in the Albany
area was scrutinized. The conclusion reached was that the increase resulted from changes in ascertainment due to changes in methods and
criteria for diagnosis (Spooner et al., 1988). The same conclusion should
obtain for other defects in both population and family studies.

There are not only striking differences in familial recurrence risk
data between centers, but within the same center. As mentioned earlier,
Emanuel and coworkers (1983) found, as did we, a substantial increase in
recurrence risk for ECD in later stages of data intake. Some of the very

lowest and very highest sib recurrence risks for different congenital heart defects have come from the same center (Anderson and Pierpont at the University of Minnesota).

Thus, large differences in sib and offspring recurrence rates could relate partially to ascertainment, partially to outliers in which a few high-risk families skew the data, and partially to the combination of several modes of inheritance under the rubric of multifactorial inheritance. Although we continue to feel that multifactorial inheritance accounts for the majority of familial cases, we have for over a decade stressed that even within multifactorial inheritance, a model that accommodates significant dominance must be considered. Mendelian, chromosomal, and even mitochondrial inheritance (Nora and Nora, 1987), genomic imprinting, and germline mosaicism may all eventually have to be entered into etiologic equations. The genetic-environmental interaction as visualized in multifactorial inheritance is not a static complex of mathematical manipulations, but is an open invitation to investigate the environmental contributions to CHD— as will be discussed in the next chapter.

When a relatively common lesion is present in 2 first-degree relatives, the empiric risk is increased on the order of 2–3 times. If it is present in 3 first-degree relatives, the risk becomes very high, either because one is dealing with a true mendelian disorder (mitochondrial inheritance) or because a highly unfavorable genetic-environmental interaction exists (type C family) within the mode of multifactorial inheritance. It is even possible that parental imprinting via transgene methylation (Swain et al., 1988) and other mechanisms may eventually be demonstrated to play a role in maldevelopment of various systems (including the cardiovascular). Preliminary findings from studies of myotonic dystrophy, Huntington's disease (Solter, 1988), cystic fibrosis (Voss et al., 1989), and retinoblastoma/osteosarcoma (Toguchida, 1989) point in this direction.

Risks in multifactorial inheritance that appear to exceed even mendelian expectation may be looked at in terms of the relationship of the distribution curve to the threshold (see Fig. 4-1). There does not appear to be disease in either parent in the family in Figure 4-2. However, knowing the natural history of VSD, it is within the realm of possibility that both parents have had VSDs that closed spontaneously in infancy or childhood. Therefore, their curve of genetic predisposition would be moved much farther to the right.

Another example, the family in Figure 4-3, is too loaded with ASDs to permit us to offer a relatively low multifactorial recurrence risk. We know that dominant inheritance is not uncommon in ASD. Therefore we counsel a high risk (50%).

A mother who must continue to take lithium to function outside of an institution cannot be told that Ebstein anomaly rarely recurs. Recurrence is not rare at all if a mother is taking lithium. There is a 10% recurrence risk of cardiac maldevelopment, most commonly Ebstein anomaly (see Chapter 5).

The child with PS and a few stigmata of Noonan syndrome, whose mother also has some subtle features of the syndrome, represents an entirely different counseling problem than a child who has no syndromic features. The difference is simply that one is dealing with high-risk dominant inheritance, not lower risk multifactorial inheritance.

These are just four examples of the need for specificity in counseling. Our present position is that empiric risks and theoretic risks have their place as very general and imprecise guidelines. The responsibility of the counselor is to be certain that he or she is as specific as the state of the art permits, and bases advice on all available clinical and historical data from the family—as well as the literature.

REFERENCES

Anderson, R.C. (1976). *Am. J. Cardiol.* **38**, 218.

Boughman, J.A., Berg, K.A., Astemborski, J.A., Clark, E.B., McCarter, R.J., Rubin, J.D., and Ferencz, C. (1987). *Am. J. Med. Genet.* **26**, 839.

Carlgren, L.E. (1959). *Br. Heart J.* **21**, 40.

Chinn, A., Fitzsimmons, J., Shepard, T.H., and Fantel, A.G. (1989). *Teratology.* **40**, 475.

Clark, E.B. (1986). In: Pierpont, M.E.M., and Moller, J.H. (eds.). *Genetics of Cardiovascular Disease.* Martinus Nijhoff Publishing, Boston. pp. 3–11.

Czeizel, A., Pornoi, A., Peterfy, E., and Tarcol, E. (1982). *Br. Heart J.* **47**, 290.

Dennis, N.R., and Warren, J. (1981). *J. Med. Genet.* **18**, 8.

Donegan, C.C., Moore, M.M., and Wiley, T.M. (1968). *Am. Heart J.* **75**, 375.

Edwards, J.H. (1969). *Br. Med. Bull.* **25**, 58.

Edwards, J.H. (1989). *Ann. Hum. Genet.* **53**, 33.

Emanuel, R., Nichols, J., and Anders, J.M. (1968). *Br. Heart J.* **49**, 144.

Emanuel, R., Somerville, J., Inns, A., and Withers, R. (1983). *Br. Heart J.* **49**, 144.

Falconer, D.S. (1965). *Ann. Hum. Genet.* **29**, 51.

Ferencz, C., Rubin, R.D., McCarter, R.J., Brenner, J.I., Neill, C.A., Perry, L.W., Hepner, S.I., and Downing, J.W. (1985). *Am. J. Epidemiol.* **121**, 31.

Ferencz, C. (1986). *Am. J. Cardiol.* **111**, 1212.

Fraser, F.C., and Hunter, A.D.W. (1975). *Am. J. Cardiol.* **36**, 793.

Fuhrmann, W. (1968). *Humangenetik.* **6**, 148.

Furhmann, W., Vogel, F. (1969). *Genetic Counseling.* Springer-Verlag, New York.

Fyler, D.C. (1980). *Pediatrics.* **65** (suppl.), 375.

Glauser, T.A., et al. (1990). *Pediatrics.* **85**, 984.

Hall, J.G., and Edwards, J.H. (1989). *Am. J. Hum. Genet.* **45** (suppl.), A48.

Hoffman, J.I.E., and Christianson, R. (1978). *Am. J. Cardiol.* **42**, 644.

Holmes, L.B., Rose, V., and Child, A.H. (1972). *Clinical Delineation of Birth Defects.* **XVI.** Williams & Wilkins, Baltimore, pp. 228–230.

Ikeda, T., et al. (1984). In: *Congenital Heart Diseases: Causes and Processes.* Nora, J.J., and Takao, A. (eds.). Futura Publishing Co., Mt. Kisko, N.Y. pp. 223–235.

Jorgensen, G., and Beuren, A.J. (1971). *Monatssch. Kinderheilkd.* **119**, 417.

Kirby, M.L. (1987). *Pediatr. Res.* **21,** 219.

Kirby, M.L. (1988). *Third Symposium on Etiology of Congenital Heart Disease.* Tokyo. Pp. 41–42.

Knoll, J.H.M., et al. (1989). *Am. J. Med. Genet.* **32,** 285.

Laursen, H.B. (1980). *Acta Pediatr. Scand.* **69,** 619.

McCredie, J. (1976). *J. Neurol. Sci.* **28,** 373.

Mitchell, S.C., Korones, S.B., and Berendes, H.W. (1971). *Circulation.* **43,** 323.

Mori, K., Ando, M., and Takao, A. (1973). *Jpn. Circulation J.* **37,** 35.

Morris, C.D., Outcalt, J., and Menashe, V.D. (1990). *Pediatrics.* **85,** 977.

Morton, N.E., Yee, S., and Elston, R.C. (1970). *Clin. Genet.* **1,** 81.

Nora, J.J. (1968a). *Circulation.* **38,** 604.

Nora, J.J., and Meyer, T.C. (1966). *Pediatrics.* **37,** 329.

Nora, J.J., and Nora, A.H. (1978a). *Circulation.* **57,** 205.

Nora, J.J., and Nora, A.H. (1978b). *Genetics and Counseling in Cardiovascular Diseases.* Charles C. Thomas, Springfield.

Nora, J.J., and Nora, A.H. (1983). *Progress in Medical Genetics.* **V.** W.B. Saunders Co., Philadelphia. pp. 91–137.

Nora, J.J., and Nora, A.H. (1987). *Am. J. Cardiol.* **59,** 459.

Nora, J.J., and Nora, A.H. (1988). *Am. J. Med. Genet.* **29,** 137.

Nora, J.J., Nora, A.H., Blu, J., Ingram, J., Fountain, A., Peterson, M., Lortscher, R.M., and Kimberling, W.J. (1978c). *JAMA.* **240,** 837.

Nora, J.J., Sommerville, R.J., and Fraser, F.C. (1968b). *Teratology.* **1,** 413.

Oakley, G.P., James, L.M., and Edmonds, L.D. (1983). *MMWR.* **32,** 755.

Okamoto, N., et al. (1984). In: *Congenital Heart Diseases: Causes and Processes.* Nora, J.J., and Takao, A. (eds.). Futura Publishing Co., Mt. Kisko, N.Y. pp. 199–231.

Pexieder, T. (1988). *Third Symposium on Etiology of Congenital Heart Disease.* Tokyo. pp. 103–104.

Pierpont, M.E.M., Gobel, J.W., Moller, J.H., and Edwards, J.E. (1988). *Am. J. Cardiol.* **61,** 423.

Rose, V., Gold, R.J.N., Lindsay, G., and Allen, M. (1985). *J. Am. Coll. Cardiol.* **6,** 376.

Sanchez-Cascos, A. (1978). *Eur. J. Cardiol.* **7,** 197.

Shimizu, T., Takao, A., Ando, M., and Hiriyama, A. (1984). In: *Congenital Heart Diseases: Causes and Processes.* Nora, J.J., and Takao, A. (eds.). Futura Publishing Co., Mt. Kisko, N.Y. pp. 29–41.

Shokeir, M.H.K. (1971). *Clin. Genet.* **2,** 7.

Smith, C. (1971). *Am. J. Hum. Genet.* **23,** 578.

Solter, D. (1988). *Ann. Rev. Genet.* **22,** 127.

Spooner, E.W., Hook, E.B., Farina, M.A., and Shaker, R.M. (1988). *Teratology.* **37,** 21.

Swain, J.L., Stewart, T.A., and Leder, P. (1988). *Cell.* **50,** 719.

Taussig, H.G., Crocetti, A., and Eshagh, E. (1971). *Johns Hopkins Med. J.* **129,** 243.

Toguchida, J. (1989). *Nature.* **338,** 156.

Voss, R., et al. (1989). *Am. J. Hum. Genet.* **45,** 313.

Weatherall, J.A. C. (ed.). (1983). EUROCAT report—*Registration of Congenital Abnormalities and Multiple Births.* No. 6, January–December, 1982, Brussels.

Whittemore, R., Hobbins, J.C., and Engle, M.A. (1982). *Am. J. Cardiol.* **50,** 641.

Williamson, E.M. (1969). *J. Med. Genet.* **6,** 255.

Yerushalmy, J. (1970). Fraser, F.C., and McKusick, V.A. (eds.). *Congenital Malformations.* Excerpta Medica, New York. p. 299.

Zetterquist, P. (1972). *A clinical and genetic study of congenital heart defects.* Thesis, Institute for Medical Genetics of the University of Uppsala, Sweden.

Zoethout, H.E., Bonham-Carter, R.E., and Carter, C.O. (1964). *J. Med. Genet.* **1,** 2.

5

Congenital Heart Disease: Environmental Factors

It is unlikely that there are many unidentified agents in our environment capable of causing the devastating teratogenesis of thalidomide (Lenz and Knapp, 1962) or rubella virus (Sever, 1970). There are likely to be many agents, however, which produce malformations in only a small percentage of exposures. But taken in aggregate, these agents may be responsible for more maldevelopment than either thalidomide or rubella. For example, if a cardiovascular teratogen is in such common use that there are exposures in 300,000 pregnancies per year, then a risk as small as 1% could produce 3,000 infants with congenital heart diseases annually. Scores of such agents may be subject to epidemiologic identification.

In this chapter we will look at some agents suspected of contributing to cardiovascular maldevelopment. Thalidomide and rubella are probably not truly representative of cardiovascular teratogens in general, in that they may require little genetic predisposition and are capable of causing such a high frequency of maldevelopment (in 50% or more of exposures during vulnerable periods of development). We have not been able to elicit a positive family history to patent ductus arteriosus (PDA) or peripheral pulmonary artery stenosis (PPAS) in infants with these abnormalities as part of their rubella syndrome. Yet even with so potent a teratogen as rubella, some genetic predisposition operates; we did find positive family histories to intracardiac defects and deafness.

Essential components to the production of an anomaly by a teratogen are:

1. Genetic predisposition
   a. to one or more forms of maldevelopment
   b. to react adversely to one or more teratogens
2. Exposure to the teratogen at a vulnerable period of embryogenesis.

There also may be many agents which are of little consequence to the population in general, but may be of grave consequence to individual families or groups with an unusual genetic predisposition.

Considerable precedence for this concept exists in the developing discipline of pharmacogenetics. There is inherited variation in susceptibility and resistance to environmental agents (Berg, 1979). The point here is that in obtaining the genetic and teratogenic history in a family with a patient having a cardiovascular anomaly, it seems entirely appropriate to counsel avoidance of nonessential agents to which there has been documented maternal exposure during cardiogenesis in an affected offspring. In fact, as a general rule, elimination of exposure to all drugs which can be safely avoided during pregnancy should be encouraged.

Certain environmental risks to humans have been selected for further discussion. A very large number of agents have been suspected because they produce malformations in animal models. However, documentation in humans is the definitive criterion that a teratogen malforms humans. Examples that illustrate the need for precise human studies are: while thalidomide is catastrophic in humans, it fails to malform many commonly used test animals and; although cortisone is a good agent to produce cleft palate in a certain strain of mouse, it does not cause cleft palate in the human.

Table 5-1 provides a general timetable we have developed from various sources for teratogenic activity in human cardiovascular structural abnormalities. Limits will vary with the teratogenic agent. For example, thalidomide appears to act within a much narrower range than rubella virus. We also know that although the usual time for spontaneous closure of the ventricular septum is 44 days postconception, spontaneous closure is not uncommon in infancy and occasionally occurs at later ages in childhood and even in early adult life. Conversely, it is difficult to visualize how truncus arteriosus, transposition of the great arteries, tetralogy of Fallot, double outlet right ventricle and other conotruncal malformations can occur after conotruncal septation is completed at 34 days after conception. Therefore, the vulnerable period for maldevelopment of these structures should be firm. A corollary of this observation is that, if a patient has a conotruncal anomaly related to a teratogen, one should look for the exposure very early in pregnancy. The treacherous aspect of this problem is that the exposure is likely to take place at a time when the mother is only just becoming aware that she is pregnant.

Table 5-1 Presumed vulnerable period for teratogenic influence on cardiovascular development

Abnormality	Embryonic event completed (days)	Limits of vulnerable period (days)	Most sensitive vulnerable period (days)
Truncoconal septation	34	14–34	18–29
Endocardial cushions	38	14–38	18–33
Ventricular septum	38–44	14–?	18–39
Atrial septum secundum	55	14–?	18–50
Semilunar valves	55	14–?	18–50
Ductus arteriosus	—	14–?	18–60
Coarctation of aorta	—	14–?	18–60

Although rubella virus has not been implicated in the production of POA in exposures later than the second trimester, there is no reason that an environmental agent could not cause persistent patency later in pregnancy. In fact, ministrations such as intravenous fluids that premature infants receive in intensive care nurseries illustrate how the postnatal environment may contribute to persistent patency of the ductus. Peripheral pulmonary artery stenosis (secondary to rubella) and aortic stenosis (secondary to type IIa homozygous hyperlipoproteinemia) are examples of structural lesions that progress after birth. We would infer that certain agents could also act on semilunar and atrioventricular valves, and systemic and pulmonary arteries in later trimesters of intrauterine life. The concept of vulnerable periods is useful when applied to some structures and related to certain teratogens, but is not inviolable.

One point to keep in mind in this chapter is that most of the environmental agents singled out for discussion require interaction with a genetic predisposition. With the exceptions of rubella virus, thalidomide, and possibly alcohol, maternal exposures to environmental teratogens at the vulnerable period of embryogenesis will not lead to maldevelopment in the majority of cases. As for cardiovascular anomalies, some agents, such as rubella, are clearly higher risk than others, such as hydantoin.

Another point that we clinicians find useful is something that may be obscured in population studies—the value of unusual patterns of subgroups of anomalies. The multiple anomalies in the thalidomide syndrome was not what called attention to the teratogen. It was the increase in frequency of the rare anomaly, phocomelia. A moderate increase in congenital malformations was not the tip-off on the teratogenicity of lithium. It was that the heart was disproportionately attacked, and that a relatively rare defect, Ebstein anomaly, was the lesion most often associated with lithium exposure (Nora et al., 1974b). Although it is perhaps useful for epidemiologists to debate whether it is anticonvulsants or epilepsy itself that is teratogenic, the clinician is able to distinguish differences in the pattern of anomalies for trimethadione as opposed to hydantoin.

The alert practitioner has been, and will continue to be, the major resource in the recognition of teratogens.

DRUGS

Alcohol

From 1900 to 1910, several reports were published concerning the increased frequency of stillbirths, infant mortality and prematurity, decreased birthweight, and retardation of growth and psychomotor development in infants of alcoholic mothers. In 1950, malformations were described as associated findings. A larger series of 127 patients was presented (Lemoise et al., 1967) in which there was a 25% frequency of malformations, most often cardiovascular defects, and cleft lip and palate.

In an effort to provide the framework for a pattern of anomalies, Jones and coworkers (1975) suggested the term fetal alcohol syndrome, which synthesized the earlier observations of other investigators with their own findings. Growth and developmental retardation, tremulousness, hyperactivity, distractibility, craniofacial (microcephaly, short palpebral fissures, short nose, and thin upper lip are prominent features) (see Fig. 5-1), joint, and cardiovascular anomalies. Cardiovascular abnormalities are present in approximately 40% of infants with *complete* fetal alcohol syndrome. These abnormalities include ventricular septal defect (the majority of cases), PDA, atrial septal defects, and other common lesions (see Table 5-2). The frequency and severity of the complete syndrome, as well as the frequency of cardiovascular anomalies, may be less if the maternal alcohol consumption is below the level of alcoholism.

The risk of damage to the fetus is as high as 50% in severe chronic alcoholics. Subtle signs may be found in the offspring of social drinkers (Hanson et al., 1978). There is evidence that even an occasional binge may be harmful. Even 10 grams of alcohol (one drink) a day may produce a detectable reduction in birth weight (Ciba Symposium, 1983). The frequency of the full blown fetal alcohol syndrome is 1 or 2 per thousand in the United States and 1 in 300 babies may show some findings.

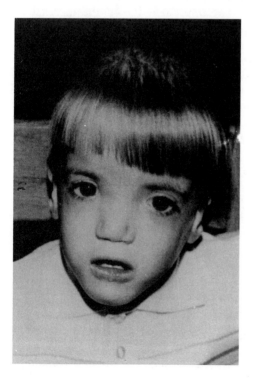

Figure 5-1 Typical facial features in fetal alcohol syndrome. Note small palpebral fissures.

Table 5-2   Selection of cardiovascular (CV) teratogens and the frequency with which CV disease is associated

Potential Teratogens	Frequency of CV disease (%)	Most common malformations
Drugs		
Alcohol (in fetal alcohol syndrome)	≈40	Ventricular septal defect (VSD), patent ductus arteriosis (PDA), atrial septal defect (ASD)
Amphetamines	≈10	VSD, PDA, ASD, transposition of the great arteries (TGA)
Anticonvulsants		
Hydantoin	2–5	Pulmonary stenosis (PS), aortic stenosis (AS), coarctation of aorta, PDA
Trimethadione	15–30	TGA,tetralogy, hypoplastic left heart
Valproic acid	>5	
Lithium	≈5	Ebstein,tricuspid atresia, ASD
Retinoic acid	15–20	VSD, ASD, PDA
Sex hormones	2–4	VSD, TGA, tetralogy
Thalidomide	5–10	Tetralogy, VSD, ASD
Infections		
Rubella	35	Peripheral pulmonary artery stenosis, PDA, VSD, ASD
Maternal conditions		
Diabetes	3–5 (30–50)	Conotruncal, VSD (for cardiomegaly and cardiomyopathy)
Lupus	≈40	Heart block
Phenylketonuria	25–100	Tetralogy, VSD, ASD

Amphetamines

Our interest in the environmental causes of cardiovascular anomalies began with a cluster of patients in a two-week period of time—three mothers who had first-trimester exposures to amphetamines delivered infants with transposition of the great arteries. We began retrospective and prospective epidemiologic studies, and animal experiments. The animal work was completed first and revealed that amphetamines were potent teratogens in animal models (Nora et al., 1965). The first retrospective study in humans involved probands up to two years of age and, while suggesting a trend, did not reveal a statistically significant difference between those mothers with amphetamine exposures and the control group (Nora et al., 1967).

The prospective study involved an obstetrical practice in which amphetamines were used almost routinely for weight control from the beginning of pregnancy. However, when the obstetricians in the practice discovered that the drug we were interested in was amphetamine, they immediately stopped prescribing it and lost interest in our having further access to their records.

We continued our retrospective study, but enrolled only probands of less than one year of age to reduce the problem of maternal memory bias. Our experience in obtaining teratogenic histories had convinced us that the older the proband, the less likely the mother would be to remember necessary details of exposures to drugs. Concentrating on histories obtained on probands in the first weeks and months of life, a statistically significant difference in amphetamine exposure was recognized in the congenital heart patients as compared with normal infants (Nora et al., 1970). Other investigators have found various malformations in the offspring of amphetamine-exposed mothers (Levin, 1971; Nelson and Forfar, 1971). Some researchers have found no increase in malformation following amphetamine exposure.

Recent data from Switzerland (Pexieder, 1989) determined a 10.9% risk of congenital cardiac disease following maternal dextroamphetamine exposure with a high relative risk of 19.6 (almost as high as for retinoic acid, and exactly as high as for heart defects following thalidomide). The common heart lesions associated with amphetamine exposure are ventricular septal defect, atrial septal defect, patent ductus arteriosus, coarctation of the aorta, and transposition of the great arteries.

Anticonvulsants

As is usually the case when discovering a human teratogen, an alert practitioner recognizes an association before large surveillance studies and monitoring centers look at accumulated data for eventual confirmation. Meadow (1968) reported the increased risk of malformations, particularly cleft lip and palate, congenital heart disease, and digital hypoplasia, (see Fig. 5-2) to offspring of epileptic mothers on anticonvulsants.

A large number of practitioner reports followed, and eventually the data from the collaborative perinatal study were analyzed and reported for the association of diphenylhydantoin and selected malformations (Monson et al., 1973). Another large survey in Czechoslovakia (Kucera, 1971) reported a marginal increase in cleft lip and palate and congenital heart disease in mothers taking anticonvulsants. Then, in 1976, the perinatal study group in conjunction with a Finnish group retracted the finding that it was diphenylhydantoin that was associated with malformations (Shapiro et al., 1976). They concluded that it was the parental epilepsy that was responsible and not the anticonvulsants.

As mentioned earlier in this chapter, the clinician has an advantage over the epidemiologist by being able to look at patterns of anomalies following a teratogenic exposure. The "Mr. Spock eyebrows," in association with other craniofacial anomalies such as mental retardation, congenital heart

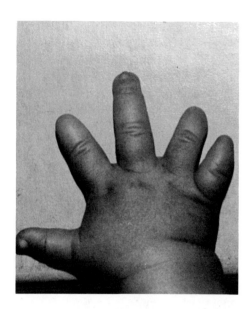

Figure 5-2 Distal digital hypoplasia associated with fetal hydantoin syndrome.

disease, and genitourinary abnormalities, is characteristic of trimethadione exposure. The multiple anomalies of many systems (including the fully developed vertebral, anal, cardiac, tracheo-esophageal, renal, and limb (VACTERL) syndrome) that have the additional finding of hypoplasia of the distal phalanges and nails points more to hydantoin. Obviously, the confounding variable of epilepsy cannot be removed, and an interaction of maternal disease with administered drugs is a valid mechanism. However, the patterns of malformation suggest to us that the drugs themselves play an important role in the maldevelopment of the fetus. Indeed, few would now dispute that several different anticonvulsants are teratogenic.

The frequency of cardiovascular disease following trimethadione exposure may be as high as 15–30% (German et al., 1970). Transposition of the great arteries, tetralogy of Fallot, and hypoplastic left heart have been reported. Valproic acid is prominently associated with neural tube defects, but congenital heart diseases have also been frequently reported and this drug appears to be slightly more teratogenic than hydantoin. Following hydantoin exposure (with and without phenobarbital), the risk of congenital heart disease has been reported to be on the order of 2–5%—most commonly pulmonary and aortic stenosis, coarctation of the aorta, and PDA. Barbiturates carry a lower risk (Pexieder, 1989). Other anticonvulsants such as carbamazepine and primidone, alone or in combination, have appeared in case reports and series.

The teratogenicity of some anticonvulsants and other drugs is associated with metabolites that are eliminated by the enzyme epoxide hydrolase. A preliminary study (Buehler et al., 1990) suggests that this enzyme may be used as a biomarker for prenatal detection of risk of the fetal hydantoin syndrome.

Aspirin

Aspirin has not been strongly implicated as a teratogen in cardiovascular maldevelopment and indeed has been exonerated in one study (Werler et al., 1989). There is a current trend to use aspirin to prevent pregnancy-induced hypertension. Theoretical risks for fetal hemorrhage remain a concern, but as of this writing, neither an increased risk of hemorrhage or an adverse influence on the ductus arteriosus has been shown in prospective studies (Schiff et al., 1989).

Attempted Abortion

The frequency of attempted abortion by consumption of drugs was probably underestimated during the years before legalized abortion in many countries. It was not uncommon that a newborn with multiple congenital anomalies, including involvement of the cardiovascular system, was the firstborn child of a young mother who was unwed or who was married after conception. On the basis of a confident physician/patient interaction, the history of attempted abortion with a variety of drugs has been disclosed. Quinine is a common agent but has been only weakly implicated as a specific trigger in maldevelopment. In an etiologic study of the Poland syndrome, there have been histories of attempted abortion (David, 1972).

Cocaine and Marijuana

Data are now accumulating which show that cocaine and marijuana are responsible for growth and neurologic impairment in the developing fetus.

The issue of cocaine and structural maldevelopment is appearing in the literature (Bingol et al., 1987; Hoyme et al., 1990) and has been discussed at national and international meetings. The evidence shows that cocaine may indeed play a role in congenital structural anomalies of the limbs, genitourinary and gastrointestinal tracts, and that vascular disruption is a mechanism. Documented but as yet unpublished, is an etiologic association with cardiovascular anomalies which occurs in the context of knowing the serious consequences to the heart and blood vessels of abusers of this drug (Virmani et al., 1988; Lange et al., 1989), the cardiovascular effects on fetal lambs, and the decreased cardiac output in infants of mothers who have abused cocaine (van de Bor et al., 1990).

We often err in the legal sense of requiring "innocent until proved guilty" for drugs like cocaine and marijuana. Data on both of these drugs, however, is convincing with regard to fetal growth (Zuckerman et al., 1989), although an etiologic association with structural anomalies has not yet been demonstrated following marijuana usage. The monitoring of pregnant women through urine specimens rather than simply through history-taking reveals a substantially higher exposure to illicit drugs than previously recognized. The potential for birth defects is, of course, only one of many risks related to drug abuse. The physician does not have to weigh prenatal risk/benefit ratios in counseling against their use.

Lithium

This agent is now a key medication in the treatment of manic-depressive psychoses and was for a time popularized in the public mind by the acclaim it had received from individual users in the entertainment world. Our suspicions regarding the teratogenic potential of lithium were aroused when we found a second patient within a period of two years who gave birth to an infant with Ebstein anomaly of the tricuspid valve following a documented exposure to the drug early in pregnancy. We reviewed the teratogenic histories we had obtained during this time period and found that in 733 histories there were only two maternal exposures to lithium; the results of both pregnancies were infants with the relatively rare Ebstein anomaly (Nora et al., 1974b). Our next step was to examine the world literature on the subject. We found there was a registry of patients who had taken lithium during pregnancy. A report from the registry had concluded that the nine infants with major malformations in 118 newborns did not represent a significant increase in anomalies over expectation in the general population (Schou et al., 1973). What was not fully appreciated was that six of the 118 infants had cardiovascular defects (a 5-fold increase over expectation) and that two of their infants had Ebstein anomaly (a 400-fold increase). With our two cases, four of 120 lithium-exposed infants had Ebstein anomaly. A subsequent report from the registry utilizing our cases and review, revealed that eleven of 143 newborns had cardiovascular anomalies (Weinstein and Goldfield, 1975). We have five patients with maternal lithium exposure and cardiovascular disease.

These data bring together an unusual anomaly and a rare exposure in pregnant women—what we have called a "Baconion exception." Phocomelia with thalidomide is a classic example. Under these circumstances, a retrospective study can be relied on to provide data of higher specificity than in the usual association of a common malformation (e.g., ventricular septal defect) with a common exposure (e.g., hormones).

Because lithium is in wide use, we feel it is important to emphasize that our assessment of the evidence leads us to believe that this drug is a potent cardiovascular teratogen in susceptible individuals and carries about a 10% risk of cardiac malformation. In our own patients, decisions regarding future exposure vary. Some mothers have stopped taking lithium and will be certain they do not take it during a future pregnancy. Others continue to take lithium, recognizing that they would not be able to function in an outpatient setting without this drug. Among these, some have made a decision against future pregnancies. Some have elected to continue their pregnancies under careful echocardiographic monitoring of the fetal heart —which may be quite informative in the proper hands.

Propranolol

Propranolol, a beta-adrenergic blocker, is used in a number of conditions such as hypertension, hypertrophic cardiomyopathy, thyrotoxicosis, and various cardiac arrhythmias. We are not familiar with any reports of cardiovascular maldevelopment resulting from maternal usage of the drug. However, bradycardia may be present in the fetus and newborn of a mother taking the drug in the final weeks of pregnancy (Gladstone et al., 1975) but the bradycardia follows a sinus mechanism and is not usually due to complete heart block (in contrast to the situation in maternal lupus). A pregnancy in a mother taking propranolol is high-risk on several counts. The newborn, in addition to having bradycardia, may be small for gestational age and hypoglycemic. Beta-adrenergic stimulation and vigorous treatment of the hypoglycemia may be required.

Retinoic Acid and Other Vitamin A Products

Retinoic acid (Accutane) is a precursor of vitamin A used orally as a treatment for severe cystic acne. Enough cases have been reported of exposure to the drug in pregnancy (Miller, 1987) to suggest risk figures as high as 40% for some type or combination of anomalies, almost half of which include cardiac maldevelopment. Etretinate is another vitamin A analogue (used for psoriasis). Case reports are appearing that also implicate this drug in birth defects, but a prospective study has not revealed cardiovascular maldevelopment (Pexieder, 1989). A few case reports of genitourinary and skeletal anomalies have been reported in hypervitaminosis A. Topical analogues (e.g., Retin-A) used for acne have not been demonstrated to be teratogenic.

Sex Hormones, Exogenous

The association of cardiac and other birth defects with exogenous sex hormones has generated a great deal of debate, which is understandable given the potential usefulness of the medications, the potential monetary value to the pharmaceutical industry, and the potential harm of drugs widely used in pregnancy if they are teratogenic. One need only recall the problems associated with stilbestrol used to prevent miscarriages.

A major use of progestogens and estrogens in the 1960s and early 1970s was as a pregnancy test. Because of data developed by several groups, including ours, this high-dose hormonal insult in the most vulnerable period of organogenesis has been abolished. Other high-dose interventions (used to maintain pregnancies and as high-dose oral contraceptives) have also been withdrawn. It is predictable, but not known on the basis of recent studies, that lower doses of exogenous hormones should be accompanied by reduced potential for teratogenicity.

Masculinization of the fetus has been recognized for 3 decades as a consequence of maternal exposure to progestogens and estrogens (Wilkins, 1960). Neural tube defects were first described by Gal et al. (1967).

Independently and almost simultaneously, Fraser and coworkers in Montreal (Levy et al., 1973) and our group in Denver (Nora and Nora, 1973) reported cardiovascular anomalies following maternal exposure to these exogenous hormones. Both groups were following personal observations and the lead of Mitchell et al. (1971) in the perinatal collaborative study who recognized an increase in transposition of the great arteries in mothers who were recorded as having maternal estrogen deficiency. Fraser's group studied various forms of transposition and found exogenous hormone exposure significantly higher in patients with these particular cardiovascular anomalies than in matched controls with mendelian disorders.

Our group has carried out three retrospective studies of cardiovascular anomalies, a prospective study, and a study of hormonal exposure in the VACTERL syndrome, which appears to be frequently associated with a number of different teratogens. In one of our three retrospective studies, infants under one year of age who had congenital heart defects of various types were matched with controls with genetic disorders. We found a significant difference for female hormone exposure. In the VACTERL syndrome study (Nora and Nora, 1975), patients were matched with four different control groups and we found highly significant differences. In a prospective study we found a two- to four-fold increase in anomalies in the infants of hormone exposed mothers. The common cardiovascular abnormalities were ventricular septal defect, transposition of the great arteries, and tetralogy of Fallot (Nora et al., 1978).

The perinatal collaborative study revealed a risk of congenital heart disease 2.3 times as high in the maternal exogenous sex hormone-exposed group as compared with those not exposed to these agents (Heinonen et al., 1977). Janerich and coworkers (1974) found an increased risk of limb reduction anomalies. A number of other studies have confirmed the association of hormones with birth defects, while several studies have failed to identify this. Many of the so-called negative studies have actually been critiques of the positive studies rather than investigations providing new data.

The question as to whether or not the current low-dose hormonal therapies used today are as teratogenic as were the hormonal pregnancy tests and high-dose therapies of previous decades is not resolved in the absence of contemporary studies. Our best guess, however, is that present hormone therapy is safer.

Thalidomide

Thalidomide had been on the market for over four years before its teratogenic potential was sufficiently documented to require its withdrawal (Lenz and Knapp, 1962). The lessons are clear. Constant vigilance is necessary to identify promptly new teratogens entering the environment. If an agent that malforms in 50–80% of exposures in the vulnerable period of structural development, including the production of a rare sentinel anomaly (phocomelia) takes four years to be indicted, how much more difficult is the task to recognize "garden variety" teratogens which cause "garden variety" malformations in only a small percentage of exposures. It was not until 1981 that the mechanism of thalidomide teratogenesis was proposed to be through a reactive intermediate, a toxic arene oxide metabolite (Gordon, 1981).

What was eventually learned from the thalidomide disaster has served as a model for our understanding of human maldevelopment caused by environmental agents in general. A timetable was developed that related the types of malformations to the period of exposure. For the heart it appeared that the exposure to produce a malformation must occur one to two weeks before the completion of the embryologic event. For example, conotruncal septation is complete by day 34 of conceptional age. There is no record in the series of Lenz (1964) or other investigators of a conotruncal abnormality following an exposure later than 29 days postconception. Conversely, no malformation occurred if exposures were before day 20. A fairly narrow sensitive period for thalidomide was calculated for defects of the heart and other structures at between 20 and 36 days after conception.

It is obvious that other environmental agents have longer periods in which they have a teratogenic influence. However, as described in the introductory portion of this chapter, teratogenic influence on most intracardiac development (exclusive of valves) should take place within the fairly short time period of about 28 days during which this phase of cardiogenesis takes place. Late-closing ventricular septal defects may be an exception.

GENETIC PREDISPOSITION TO TERATOGENS

One need only glance through the *Physicians Desk Reference* to appreciate the caution that drug companies are at last using to warn against taking almost any drug during the first trimester of pregnancy. And the *Catalog of Teratogenic Agents* has over 2,000 entries in which there are human or animal data or both. So the few drugs appearing in the foregoing discussion and in Table 5-2 are only some that the authors have judged to have now, or in the past, informative etiologic possibilities in cardiovascular maldevelopment as it relates to the population.

It is not unlikely that the majority of environmental agents that interact with a genetic predisposition to maldevelopment (and when given at a vulnerable period of embryogenesis) are low-risk to the broader population and require a narrow confluence of conditions to produce a birth defect in a given family. Such agents would not be easily identified in an epidemiologic study, but in taking a teratogenic history following a birth defect, these could be suspected and cautioned against in future pregnancies.

Now it is becoming possible to move from population level concepts of genetic predisposition to the cellular level and to the biochemical nature of genetic predisposition relating to environmental teratogens (mutagens and carcinogens). One such example, studied most extensively in the mouse, that has important implications for congenital heart disease in the human is the work of Nebert's group (1978, 1987). The mechanism for the clearance of many drugs and chemicals involves cytosolic receptors, phase I oxidative enzymes (e.g., the cytochrome P-450-mediated monooxygenases), reactive intermediates, and phase II conjugating enzymes. When a chemical enters the body, it has to be eliminated. Consider for example, hydrocarbons such as benzpyrene or exogenous steroid hormones. These chemicals circulate in the body, enter individual cells, and have the potential for participating in biochemical functions. There is a dynamic body chemistry for chemicals as well as for nutrients, in which there is a transformation-utilization-excretion cycle.

When there is a genetic abnormality or breakdown in the cycle, and chemicals that should be excreted accumulate, damage results. For example, aromatic hydrocarbons entering a cell form complexes with cytosolic receptors. These complexes activate the structural genes for cytochrome P-450 and other enzymes. These metabolize the chemicals to the point of their becoming reactive intermediates, such as a toxic epoxides. These epoxides have the potential to produce cellular damage ranging from carcinogenesis and mutagenesis to teratogenesis. The urgent need of the cell to maintain its integrity is met in most cases by a further step utilizing phase II enzymes to render the chemical product biologically harmless to the host and to lead to its excretion.

Some strains of mice (and families of humans) respond vigorously to the message initiated by the hydrocarbon-receptor complex to manufacture phase I enzymes to handle the chemical exposure. The strains of mice that respond vigorously by making large amounts of enzymes to handle the sudden influx of chemicals are appropriately called responders. They possess a responsive form of the gene. Other strains do not respond and are thus termed genetic nonresponders. The ability to respond is transmitted following mendelian laws. Parents may transmit the trait of responsiveness or nonresponsiveness to their offspring. To illustrate, a nonresponsive mother carrying a responsive fetus is exposed to a load of aromatic hydrocarbons. What should the outcome be? Certainly it appears to be useful for the organism to be able to biotransform chemicals in a rapid and efficient manner in preparation for excretion. Unfortunately, the responsiveness that helps an adult cope with chemicals in the environment may not be useful for a developing fetus that may only be efficient in carrying the biotransformation through phase I, but then may not be able to proceed promptly enough through its immature systems (e.g., glutathione limiting) to the second phase of detoxifying the reactive intermediates.

It is here, in the reactive intermediates, that an important potential for cellular damage lies. It should also be pointed out that body economy is obviously not without limits. Intuitively, the body is not likely to have the capacity to create an entirely new receptor to handle each new chemical that enters the environment. Drug companies may make small changes in a basic chemical structure for various reasons, and thus own the new variant. But the body is not attuned to develop entirely new biotransformation systems to take care of each new synthetic chemical variant. Rather, the cytosolic receptors may be multipotential, capable of handling related chemicals as if they were identical. There is, however, an irony in all of this. The genetic traits that help an adult escape chemical poisoning may predispose a developing fetus to birth defects, such as cardiovascular malformations.

From this brief exploration of one small portion of genetic predisposition (in this case involving major genes and thresholds), it should be clear how essential is the interaction between heredity and environment in maldevelopment. Of course, there are many mechanisms of teratogenesis that exceed the scope of this presentation. A necessary understanding in the context of what is being presented in this section is that in the early stages of development, morphogenesis is progressing so rapidly that a minor environmental stimulus can produce major maldevelopment.

INFECTIOUS AGENTS

Rubella Virus

This most devastating of teratogens was first recognized as being responsible for a triad of abnormalities: cataracts, deafness, and patent ductus arteriosus (Gregg, 1941). Over the years, and especially following the rubella pandemic of 1964–1965, a number of other anomalies were recognized and incorporated into what became known as the expanded rubella syndrome (Cooper and Krugman, 1966). Psychomotor retardation, bone and skin lesions, hepatitis, hepatosplenomegaly, anemia, purpura, glaucoma, and retinopathy were frequently found.

Our experience with a sizable series in Houston revealed that 71% of patients with the rubella syndrome acquired during the pandemic of 1964–1965 had some form of cardiovascular disease. The risk of some abnormality, in the review of Sever (1970), was 50% for an exposure in the first month, 22% in the second month, and 6–10% in the third, fourth, and fifth months. Peripheral pulmonary artery stenosis (PPAS), with or without pulmonary valve stenosis, was the most common problem and present in 55% of our patients. Patent ductus arteriosus (PDA) was present in 43% and a variety of other lesions in 8% (including ventricular septal defect, atrial septal defect, aortic stenosis, and tetralogy of Fallot). It was common for a patient to have more than one cardiovascular abnormality.

There was no positive family history of cardiovascular maldevelopment in patients with PPAS and PDA, but such a history was found in 38% of patients with other lesions. This suggested to us that the genetic contribution to PPAS and PDA was minimal, but for other cardiac malformations the genetic-environmental interaction may have been operating at a level comparable to our experience with nonrubella patients.

Immunization can essentially eradicate the threat of malformation from rubella virus if there is universal compliance and if complacency does not supervene. A question may be raised as to what role rubella virus is continuing to play in the incidence of congenital cardiovascular disease in countries and communities in which immunization is less than optimal. Does this explain part of the difference in incidence rates in conflicting studies?

Other Viruses

Several viruses in addition to rubella have been implicated in the etiology of congenital malformations of the heart. Presumptive evidences that in utero infections may play a role in a relatively high percentage of congenital heart lesions was derived from our finding of abnormal elevations of IgM and antiheart IgM in the sera of 13 of 37 newborns (35%) with congenital heart diseases (Nora et al., 1974c).

Viruses that are generally recognized as being teratogenic in man include rubella, cytomegalovirus and *herpesvirus hominis* (Blattner et al., 1973). Although congenital cardiovascular diseases clearly follow rubella infection, such an association of maternal infections with cytomegalovirus and herpes, while described, have not been well established. Coxsackie B and Asian influenza viruses have also been implicated, but there have been conflicting results. Enteroviruses appear to be related to intrauterine myocarditis, but not to structural maldevelopment. Endocardial fibroelastosis has been attributed to intrauterine infection with mumps virus and with Coxsackie B virus. This will be discussed in the next section as an immunologic consideration.

There is much to be learned regarding the influence of maternal viral infections on intrauterine development of many systems (including the cardiovascular). Informative studies are easy to propose, but difficult and expensive to perform. If and when such studies are completed, we would predict that a wide variety of viral infections in addition to rubella will be revealed as important in cardiovascular teratogenesis.

Other Infections and Immunologic Considerations

Congenital toxoplasmosis and syphilis are two nonviral infectious diseases associated with malformations in the newborn. Syphilis has not been implicated in the etiology of congenital cardiovascular disease, but toxoplasmosis has infrequently been reported with cardiomyopathy. They do,

however, serve to keep before us the possibility that bacterial and pro-
tozoan infections, by various mechanisms, have the theoretical potential
to play a role in the maldevelopment of the cardiovascular system, as well
as other systems.

Response to intrauterine infections of various types may be recognized
by an elevation of serum IgM in the newborn. A question has been raised
regarding the etiologic implications of a positive skin test to mumps in
endocardial fibroelastosis (EFE). Is this a nonspecific reaction signifying
only that an immune response exists in the infant with fibroelastosis to
shared antigen in the material used for mumps skin tests? St. Geme and
coworkers (1970) proposed that a true intrauterine mumps antigenic exposure has taken place. This may be true in some cases, but evidence is
lacking for significant intercurrent illnesses in the vast majority of pregnancies in which infants were born who eventually developed EFE.

Then what about mild infections or autoimmune disease? We have
found antiheart IgG circulating in the serum of mothers of infants with
EFE, but this occurred so frequently in our matched controls that we were
unable to discriminate between the groups on this basis. In fact, antiheart
antibody becomes more common the higher the parity of the mother.
Infants with EFE have a higher birth rank in the largest series in the
literature (Chen et al., 1971). Can antiheart antibody itself be teratogenic?
Perhaps. In one of our studies we found antiheart antibody to be more
teratogenic to the heart than antikidney antibody in the mouse, which may
suggest some specificity (Nora et al., 1974a).

Where does immunodeficiency fit into the puzzle? In DiGeorge syndrome, thymic aplasia coexists with conotruncal anomalies presumably
under the influence of neural crest disruption. Animal models illustrate
how teratogens can adversely affect the neural crest and lead to conotruncal and thymic abnormalities (Ikeda et al., 1984). A number of other
syndromes (listed in Table 7-1) also fit in the cardiofacial/neural crest
category. Immune deficiency is, in the experience of some observers,
characteristic of various nonsyndromic conotruncal anomalies, such as
tetralogy of Fallot.

It is clear that there are numerous pertinent and potentially fruitful
questions to be explored in the area of infections and immune response in
the etiology of cardiovascular maldevelopment.

MATERNAL CONDITIONS

Diabetes Mellitus

An increased rate of malformation is recognized in the children of diabetic
mothers (Lemons et al., 1981). Since these mothers frequently take hypoglycemic agents, it is difficult to separate the effects of the maternal illness
from the effects of or interactions with medications. Sulfonylurea com-

pounds and insulin have come under suspicion as teratogens. Prediabetic and gestational diabetic mothers receiving no hypoglycemic agents appear to have an increase in the frequency rate of malformed infants in some series and not in others. The amniotic fluid in diabetic women demonstrates increased mutagenic activity (Nylander Rivrud et al., 1988) which could contribute to developmental errors. This mutagenic activity is further enhanced by smoking.

The relative risk for all malformations to the offspring of insulin-dependent diabetic mothers is 7.9%, the relative risk of cardiovascular anomalies is 18%, and the absolute risk is 8.5% cardiovascular malformations of livebirths (Bacerra et al. 1990).

The so-called caudal regression syndrome (Kucera, 1971) of missing lumbosacral vertebrae and lower limb malformations has been considered a characteristic pattern in infants of diabetic mothers (IDM). However, a confounding variable is that for many years diabetic mothers were routinely given progestogens to help maintain their pregnancies.

The kinds of cardiovascular defects include structural abnormalities, predominantly conotruncal abnormalities and ventricular septal defect (Ferencz et al., 1990). A link between maternal diabetes and neural crest disruption is suggested by the higher than expected frequency of double outlet right ventricle, truncus, and other conotruncal anomalies in IDM. Another common problem is the cardiomyopathy in the newborn IDM. The echocardiographic findings may mimic those of asymmetric septal hypertrophy (ASH). Data suggest that 30–50% of newborn IDM have cardiomegaly (Wolfe and Way, 1977), 10–20% have nonobstructive cardiomyopathy, and about 5% have obstructive cardiomyopathy. This problem is reversible and echocardiography may be used to document the diminution in septal hypertrophy along with the improvement shown in the chest x-ray and the clinical course. Excluding cardiomyopathy, structural cardiac anomalies are still the most common congenital defects in the IDM, accounting for 35–42% of the malformations (Khoury et al., 1989; Bacerra et al., 1990).

Primary prevention of mortality and morbidity in IDM should be directed at the institution of precise control of insulin-dependent diabetes before conception. Perhaps similar efforts should also be directed toward women with risk factors for gestational and noninsulin-dependent diabetes.

Lupus and Other Maternal Autoimmune Diseases

Since the early reports of this condition (McCue et al., 1977), complete heart block has been observed to occur in as high as 40% of infants of mothers with systemic lupus erythematosis and similar autoimmune diseases. Discoid lupus in the newborn (Fig. 5-3) is a common finding. Fetal loss is about 30%. It is essential to monitor pregnancies for the presence of fetal bradycardia and to be prepared at the time of delivery for resuscita-

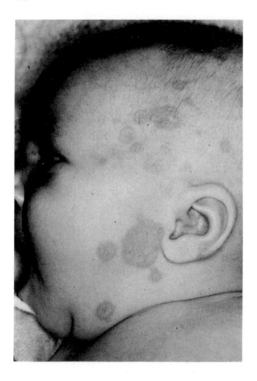

Figure 5-3 Skin lesions of discoid lupus developing two weeks after birth in infant with congenital complete heart block whose mother had systemic lupus erythematosus.

tion and the maintenance of adequate cardiac output in the newborn until his or her condition is stabilized. Once stability is achieved, the infant with complete heart block can usually be maintained without medication or a pacemaker. The heart rate, as is often the case in congenital complete heart block, is somewhat responsive to exercise. A pacemaker may be required eventually in later childhood or adult life. If attention is not aggressively directed in the immediate newborn period toward maintenance of cardiac output, death may result. Eventual restoration of a normal sinus rhythm is a theoretical possibility, but we are not familiar with reports of this happening, nor have we seen it in our small experience.

Maternal IgE antibodies to Ro (a soluble tissue ribonucleoprotein) damages the conducting system of the developing heart (Lee et al., 1983). Selective calcification within the ventricular septum has been seen at autopsy. Familial cases (Winkler et al., 1977) are now commonly recognized with a recurrence in siblings of 20–40% irrespective of the status of the maternal disease.

Phenylketonuria

Prior to the use of low phenylalanine diets, reproductive fitness in phenylketonuria was greatly impaired. During the past decade there has been an increasing awareness of the significant teratogenicity of high maternal blood levels of phenylalanine. Most of the offspring of phenylketonuric mothers and normal fathers have moderate to severe psychomotor and growth retardation, microcephaly, and other congenital anomalies. Congenital heart disease is found in as high as 25–100% of these patients, depending on which study is used (Stevenson and Huntley, 1967; Fisch et al. 1969; Pexieder, 1989). Tetralogy of Fallot and other conotruncal malformations are most common, perhaps reflecting the early timing of the teratogenic insult. Ventricular and atrial septal defects, coarctation of the aorta, and PDA have also been reported.

MISCELLANEOUS AGENTS

There are many other agents, drugs, radiation, and maternal conditions that have not been discussed for a variety of reasons. Radiation, alkylating agents, folic acid, and warfarin are clearly teratogenic, but have not been reported to malform the heart. Antibiotics, maternal thyroid conditions and exogenous thyroid, tranquilizers, and antituberculosis drugs keep appearing in the literature in case reports. Though often quite suggestive, these are still not definitive enough to bring in an indictment of cardiovascular teratogenicity. We suspect that many of such agents could be low-risk to those genetically predisposed. Bendectin may have a slightly increased relative risk, but cannot be clearly indicted. Chemical pollutants such as pesticides, industrial solvents, methyl mercury, and cigarette smoke have come under suspicion, and while some may eventually be demonstrated to be human cardiovascular teratogens, the data are still too soft to develop here.

PROBLEMS IN IDENTIFYING TERATOGENS

As mentioned earlier, even in the case of thalidomide which had a 50–80% malformation rate, more than 4 years elapsed from the time the drug appeared on the market until the data were convincing enough to require its withdrawal. How much greater is the challenge to discover low-level teratogens? But what if a drug causes malformations in only 1 or 2% of those exposed, does it really matter all that much? It matters most tragically to those who must carry the burden of disability and death, particularly if the use of the drug was not absolutely essential. From the point of view of society it also matters. If a drug is commonly used in pregnancy, then the potential exposure rate is high. And even if the malformation rate following exposure is only 1–2%, this could mean thousands of babies every year in the United States alone with birth defects that could have been prevented. Thus, to the individual's burden must be added the unnecessary and unacceptable burden to society.

A critical error that flaws many epidemiologic studies is the failure to associate the time of exposure to the teratogen with the vulnerable period of embryogenesis for the defect in question. This requirement must include cases with malformations to establish that the putative causal exposure occurred at the vulnerable period. To illustrate this point, many studies have looked at transposition of the great arteries (TGA). Conotruncal septation is completed by day 34. Any teratogenic influence on this structural development must take place before that day. Therefore, a drug given after day 34 cannot be considered responsible for TGA, nor can a case where teratogenic exposure after day 34 that failed to produce transposition be tallied as showing no effect. In our own studies we have emphasized the absolute necessity of correlation of the time of exposure with the stage of vulnerability.

The magnitude of the problem of using the full first 3 months as the vulnerable period, rather than from 2–6 weeks postconception (a 67% mismodeling bias) may not be readily apparent until one performs the appropriate calculations (Nora et al. 1982; Nora and Fraser, 1989). If one builds into a study a 67% error through mismodeling (as compared with a tolerable 5% error), the number of cases needed to show no association for a teratogen with birth defects at a 4-fold increase in risk balloons from only 140 cases to 2,299 cases needed in a retrospective study or to 12,122 cases (rather than 1,663) in a prospective study. To put it another way, 16 times as many retrospective cases are needed to show "no effect" if the first trimester rather than the one month vulnerable period is used as the true vulnerable period. What if the increase in risk is only 2-fold (as in increasing congenital defects from an incidence of 1–2% in exposed groups)? Then 60,231 cases would be required to show "no effect" in a prospective study.

Few studies can tolerate a 67% mismodeling bias. The solution seems to be self-evident. Precision in design greatly reduces the number of cases needed to reach confident conclusions. One may either have tens of thousands of cases studied imprecisely or a few hundred cases that are studied with precision. Financial resources will no longer permit the profligacy of enormous but imprecise studies. Small, elegant, well-designed studies will achieve the answers with greater economy and accuracy. Malformation registries may eventually provide the data for case-control and cohort studies large enough to elucidate teratogenic factors not detectable by sample sizes available to a single center.

The question of teratogens in human malformations may be looked at from 2 perspectives: that of the patient and his family, and that of the researcher. It is relatively easy to identify an agent as teratogenic if it produces a high frequency of an uncommon anomaly. The goal becomes even easier to reach if the agent has just been introduced or is not in widespread use. Thalidomide and lithium are examples. However, it is extremely difficult—some say almost impossible—to identify a teratogen that is widely used and causes a small increase in common anomalies. Yet as hazards to public health, the agents in the latter category can be quantitatively more important.

REFERENCES

Bacerra, J.E., Khoury, M.J., Cordero, J.F., and Erickson, J.D. (1990). *Pediatrics* **85**, 1.

Berg, K. (1979). *Genetic Damage in Man Caused by Environmental Agents.* Academic Press, New York, pp. 1–25.

Bingol, N., Fuchs, M., Diaz, V., Stone, R.K., and Gromisch, D.S. (1987). *J. Pediatr.* **110**, 93.

Blattner, R.J., Williamson, A.P., and Heys, F.M. (1973). *Prog. Med. Virol.* **15**, 1.

Buehler, B.A., Delimont, D., van Waes, M., and Finnell, R.H. 1990). *N. Engl. J. Med.* **322**, 1567.

Chen, S., Thompson, M.W., and Rose. V. (1971). *J. Pediatr.* **79**, 385.

Ciba Foundation Symposium 105. (1983). *Mechanisms of Alcohol Damage in Utero.* Porter, R., (ed). Pitman, London.

Cooper, L.Z., and Krugman, S. (1966). *Pediatrics* **37**, 335.

David, T.J. (1972). *N. Engl. J. Med.* **287**, 487.

Ferencz, C., Rubin, J.D., McCarter, R.J., and Clark, E.B. (1990). *Teratology* **41**, 319.

Fisch, R.O., Doeden, D., and Lansky, L.L. (1969). *Am. J. Dis. Child.* **118**, 847.

Gal, K., Kirman, B., and Stern, I. (1967). *Nature* **216**, 83.

German, J., Kowal, A., and Ehlers, K.H. (1970). *Teratology* **3**, 349.

Gladstone, G.R., Hardof, A., and Gersony, W.M. (1975). *J. Pediatr.* **86**, 962.

Gordon, G.B. (1981). *Proc. Natl. Acad. Sci. USA.* **78**, 2545.

Gregg, N.M. (1941). *Trans. Ophthalmol. Soc. Aust.* **3**, 35.

Hanson, J.W., Streissguth, A.P., and Smith, D.W. (1978). *J. Pediatr.* **92**, 457.

Heinonen, O.P., Slone, D., and Monson, R.R. (1977). *N. Engl. J. Med.* **296**, 67.

Hoyme, H.E. et al. (1990). *Pediatrics* **85**, 743.

Ikeda, T. et al. (1984). In: *Congenital Heart Diseases: Causes and Processes.* Nora, J.J., and Takao, A. (eds.). Futura Publishing Co., Mt. Kisko, New York. pp. 223–235.

Janerich, D.T., Piper, J.M., and Glebatis, D.M. (1974). *N. Engl. Med.* **291**, 697.

Jones, K.L., and Smith, D.W. (1975). *Teratology* **12**, 1.

Khoury, M.J., Bacerra, J.E., Cordero, J.F., and Erickson, J.D. (1989). *Pediatrics* **84**, 658.

Kucera, J. (1971). *Teratology* **4**, 492.

Lange, R.A. et al. (1989). *N. Engl. J. Med.* **321**, 1557.

Lee, L. et al. (1983). *Ann. Intern. Med.* **99**, 592.

Lemoise, P., Haroussea, H., and Borteyru, J.P. (1967). *Arch. Fr. Pediatr.* **25**, 830.

Lemons, J.A., Vargas, P., and Delaney, J.J. (1981). *Obstet. Gynecol.* **57**, 187.

Lenz, W. (1964). *Proceedings of the Second International Conference on Congenital Malformations.* The International Medical Congress Ltd., New York.

Lenz, W., and Knapp K. (1962). *Arch. Environ. Health.* **5**, 100.

Levin, J.N. (1971). *J. Pediatr.* **79**, 130.

Levy, E.P., Cohen, A., and Fraser, F.C. (1973). *Lancet.* **1**, 611.

McCue, C.M., Mantakas, M.E., and Tingelstad, J.E. (1977). *Circulation* **56**, 82.

Meadow, S.R. (1968). *Lancet* **2**, 1296.

Miller, R.K. (1987). *Teratology* **35**, 269.

Mitchell, S.C., Sellman, E.H., and Westphal, M.C. (1971). *Am. J. Cardiol.* **28**, 653.

Monson, R.R., Rosenberg, L., and Hartz, S.C. (1973). *N. Engl. J. Med.* **289**, 1048.

Nebert, D.W. (1978). *Hum. Genet. (suppl.)* **1**, 149.

Nebert, D.W., and Gozales, F.J. (1987). *Hospital Practice* **22**, 63.

Nelson, M.M., and Forfar, J.O. (1971). *Br. Med. J.* **1,** 153.

Nora, J.J. et al. (1978). *JAMA* **240,** 837.

Nora, A.H., and Nora, J.J. (1975). *Arch. Environ. Health.* **30,** 17.

Nora, J.J., and Fraser, F.C. (1989). *Medical Genetics: Principles and Practice.* 3rd ed. Lea & Febiger, Philadelphia, p. 271.

Nora, J.J., McNamara, D.G., and Fraser, F.C. (1967). *Lancet* **1,** 570.

Nora, J.J., Nihill, M.R., and Miles, V.N. (1974a). *Teratology* **9,** 143.

Nora, J.J., and Nora, A.H. (1973). *Pediatr. Res.* **7,** 321.

Nora, J.J., Nora, A.H., and Toews, W.H. (1974b). *Lancet* **2,** 594.

Nora, J.J., Nora, A.H., and Wexler, P. (1982). *Am. J. Obstet. Gynecol.* **144,** 860.

Nora, J.J., Trasler, D.G., and Fraser, F.C. (1965). *Lancet* **2,** 1021.

Nora, J.J., Vargo, T.A., and Nora, A.H. (1970). *Lancet* **1,** 1290.

Nora, J.J., Weishuhn, E.J., and Bourland, B.J. (1974c). *Br. Heart J.* **36,** 167.

Nylander Rivrud, G., Moen, M., Moe, N., Berg, K., and Bjøro, K. (1988). *Gynecol. Obstet. Invest.* **26,** 113.

Pexieder, T. (1989). *DIA-GM.* **3,** 201.

Schiff, E. et al. (1989). *N. Engl. J. Med.* **321,** 351.

Schou, M., Goldfield, M.D., and Weinstein, M.R. (1973). *Br. Med. J.* **2,** 135.

Sever, J. (1970). *Congenital Malformations.* Excerpta Medica, Amsterdam. pp. 180–186.

Shapiro, S., Hartz, S., and Siskind, V. (1976). *Lancet* **1,** 273.

Stevenson, R.E., and Huntley, C.C. (1967). *Pediatrics* **40,** 33.

St. Geme, J.W. Jr., Noren, G.R., and Evans, C.M. (1970). *Pediatrics* **46,** 134.

van de Bor, M., Walther, F.J., and Ebrahimi, M. (1990). *Pediatrics* **85,** 30.

Virmani, R., Rabinowitz, M., Smialek, J.E., and Smyth, D.F. (1988). *Am. Heart J.* **155,** 1056.

Weinstein, M.R., and Goldfield, M.D. (1975). *Am. J. Psychiatry* **132,** 529.

Werler, M.M., Mitchell, A.A., and Shapiro, S. (1989). *N. Engl. J. Med.* **321,** 1639.

Wilkins, L. (1960). *JAMA.* **172,** 1028.

Winkler, R.B., Nora, A.H., and Nora, J.J. (1977). *Circulation* **56,** 1103.

Wolfe, R.R., and Way, G.I. (1977). *Johns Hopkins Med. J.* **140,** 177.

Zuckerman, B. et al. (1989). *N. Engl. J. Med.* **320,** 762.

6

Cardiovascular Disease: Single-Gene Disorders

Many single-gene mutations produce cardiovascular disease as a feature of a syndrome (e.g., Marfan) or as a discrete abnormality (such as hypertrophic cardiomyopathy). This chapter will be divided according to the mode of inheritance. Except for MPS II, diseases that have more than one mode (such as osteogenesis imperfecta) will be located in the section that encompasses the cases that predominate (autosomal dominant for osteogenesis imperfecta). Gene localization will be mentioned for a number of mendelian syndromes, which brings up the possibility of the use of DNA markers for prenatal diagnosis. The genetics of several syndromes that have cardiovascular lesions has not been clearly established, and will be discussed in Chapter 7. Because of constraints of space it will not be possible, nor is it necessarily useful, to detail all syndromes in which cardiovascular disease has been encountered. Rather, we will briefly describe cardiovascular implications of some of the more informative and common conditions. Syndromes with structural maldevelopment and important vascular and myocardial involvement, such as homocystinuria and Fabry disease, will be discussed here. Cardiomyopathies and conduction defects of various etiologic modes, in which a syndrome is not as prominent, represent a category that is logically covered separately in Chapter 9.

The counseling for risk of recurrence of a mendelian condition is straightforward (e.g., 50% for autosomal dominant, 25% for autosomal recessive, and female carrier to 50% of male offspring for X-linked recessive). Exceptions will be noted as they occur. We have had to draw heavily from our own impressions and experience in many instances in which the literature was lacking or conflicting with respect to the frequency of cardiovascular involvement in various syndromes. Obviously we would not include syndromes in which cardiovascular disease is not an important or informative component.

As is the case in chromosomal anomalies in the etiology of cardiovascular maldevelopment, when considering single-mutant-gene causation, it is best (with a few notable exceptions) to look for a syndrome of multiple abnormalities. The format of presentation in this chapter will be to list the syndromes or discrete disorders alphabetically under each of three headings: autosomal dominant, autosomal recessive, and X-linked. There is no easy solution to the problem of alternative names for the same condition. Some people abhor eponyms. Other people may dislike inconsistencies such as using eponyms for some disorders and not for others. We have simply alphabetized the diseases in Tables 6-1, 6-2, 6-3, and in the text by the names we use.

A note must be made here regarding echocardiographic illustrations throughout this book, almost all of which are M-mode. In practice today, two dimensional (2-D, real-time) Doppler and color flow imaging are used in clinical evaluation. For measurements and for diagnostic criteria, however, we have more often selected M-mode, and for clarity of anatomic detail, we choose angiocardiographic contrast studies.

AUTOSOMAL DOMINANT CARDIOVASCULAR ABNORMALITIES

Apert Syndrome (Acrocephalosyndactyly)

The distinguishing features of this syndrome are the tall head with short anteroposterior diameter and irregular craniosynostosis, and the osseous or cutaneous syndactyly of the hands and feet (see Table 6-1 and Fig. 6-1).

Table 6-1 Selected autosomal dominant cardiovascular abnormalities

Abnormality	Types of cardiovascular disease
Apert	VSD, TOF, coarctation of aorta (CA)
Asymmetric crying facies (ACF)	Ventricular septal defect (VSD), tetralogy of Fallot (TOF)
Atrial septal defect (ASD)	(see Chapter 5)
Cardiomyopathy, hypertrophic	(see Chapter 9)
Cardiomyopathy, dilated	(see Chapter 9)
Conduction defects, familial	(see Chapter 9)
Endocardial fibroelastosis (EFE)	(see Chapter 9)
Holt-Oram	ASD, VSD
LEOPARD	Cardiomyopathy, Pulmonary stenosis (PS)
Marfan	Mitral and aortic disease
Mitral valve prolapse (MVP)	MVP, mitral insufficiency (MI)
Myotonic dystrophy (Steinert)	Conduction defects, myocardial disease
Neurofibromatosis I (NFI)	Hypertension, pulmonary stenosis (PS)
Noonan	PS, ASD, cardiomyopathy
Osler-Weber-Rendu	AV fistula, pulmonary hypertension
Osteogenesis imperfecta (OI)	MI, aortic insufficiency (AI)
Primary pulmonary hypertension	Primary pulmonary hypertension
Romano-Ward (Long Q-T)	(see Chapter 9)
Supravalvular aortic stenosis (SVAS) (with or without elfin facies)	Supravalvular aortic and pulmonary stenosis, peripheral pulmonary stenosis
Tuberous sclerosis	Myocardial rhabdomyoma and angioma
Velocardiofacial	VSD, TOF
Von Hippel-Lindau (VHL)	Hemangioma, hypertension

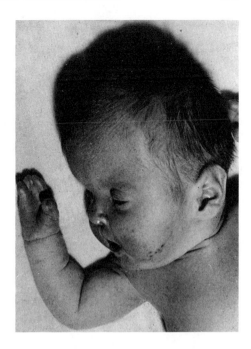

Figure 6-1 Typical head shape and "mitten hand" in infant with Apert Syndrome.

Cardiovascular abnormalities occur more frequently than in the general population, about 10% in one series (Cohen, 1972). Ventricular septal defect, tetralogy of Fallot, coarctation of the aorta, and conduction abnormalities have been found.

Asymmetric Crying Facies (Cayler Syndrome)

The first patients we saw with Cayler syndrome (Cayler, 1969) asymmetric crying facies (ACF) had tetralogy of Fallot, and we were concerned that they had sustained strokes. Studies have since shown that hypoplasia of the depressor anguli oris muscle (Nelson and Eng, 1972), not facial paralysis, is the cause of the asymmetry (see Fig. 6-2). A variety of heart defects are associated with this facial abnormality, most often ventricular septal defect, but also atrial septal defect, atrioventricular canal, single ventricle, coarctation of the aorta, and pulmonary stenosis. It appears that about 20% of individuals with ACF have some form of congenital heart disease. The evidence is now strong that ACF is autosomal dominant and the spectrum of associated abnormalities may include microcephaly, mental retardation (Silengo et al., 1986), as well as skeletal, and other visceral anomalies.

Ehlers-Danlos Syndrome (Hyperelastosis Cutis)

Considerable genetic heterogeneity exists, with at least fourteen distinct forms, seven of which are autosomal dominant, six recessive, and one

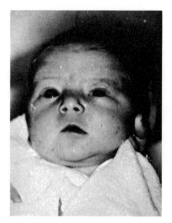 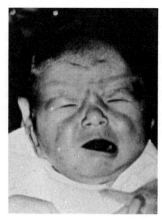

Figure 6-2   In asymmetric crying facies the feature is observable with crying (right) but is not readily apparent at rest (left).

X-linked. This disorder of connective tissue (depending on the form) manifests itself with findings of distensible fragile skin, hyperextensible joints, inguinal and umbilical hernias, and cardiovascular problems in a more extensive catalog of abnormalities (McKusick, 1972; Prockop and Kivirikko, 1984). The autosomal dominant forms are the more common, and the recognition of penetrance is influenced by the often mild expression of the diagnostic features.

The cardiovascular involvement includes structural maldevelopment of the heart, such as atrial septal defect and tetralogy of Fallot, but the vascular defects have been more traditionally emphasized. Large and medium-size arteries are affected. Dissecting aortic aneurysm and ruptures of arteries, such as subclavian, axillary, popliteal, and various cerebral vessels are dramatic and fatal events. It should be obvious that cardiac catheterization of these patients is hazardous.

Echocardiography has allowed us to appreciate how common atrioventricular valve dysfunction is in these patients. This technique provides an additional diagnostic criterion in arriving at a diagnosis of Ehlers-Danlos syndrome in individuals with borderline features. The frequency of some form of cardiovascular disease is high. A present estimate of cardiovascular risk would be greater than 50% of individuals with type IV disease (Sachs type) and somewhat less than 50% for all autosomal dominant forms.

Pregnancy represents a risk to both mother and infant. Excessive bleeding, tears, and uterine rupture occur in the mother. Bleeding, spontaneously ruptured membranes, and prematurity are threats to the fetus and newborn.

Holt-Oram Syndrome (Heart and Hand Syndrome)

There are several syndromes in which limb and heart anomalies coexist. We reserve the term Holt-Oram syndrome for the autosomal dominant transmission of the association of cardiac anomalies (most often atrial septal defect, ventricular septal defect, or both together) and upper limb anomalies (Holt and Oram, 1960; Gall et al., 1966). The limb anomalies (Fig. 6-3) vary from slight fingerization of the thumb to radial aplasia. Since there are both important genetic and environmental considerations in the etiology of syndromes involving the heart and limbs, it is essential that prior to counseling, an examination of first-degree relatives take place. If the proband is a young infant, a reliable teratogenic history may also be possible. The clues to the syndrome being Holt-Oram (and thus dominant) may be as subtle as finding in a first-degree relative a slight fingerization of a thumb or faint ejection murmur at the base, accompanied by a constantly split second sound.

LEOPARD Syndrome

This rare syndrome is included because it may reflect neural crest disruption (St. John Sutton et al., 1981), which is discussed in Chapter 4 under

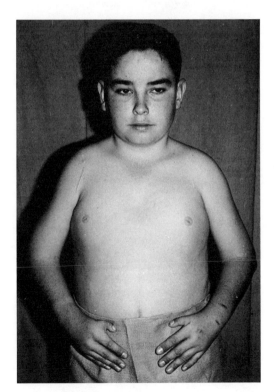

Figure 6-3 Note severe hypoplasia of thumbs in this patient with Holt-Oram syndrome who also had both an atrial septal defect and ventricular septal defect.

Pathogenesis and is illustrated by a number of conditions in Chapter 7 and listed in Table 7-1. The acronym stands for Lentigines, Electrocardiographic conduction defects, Ocular hypertelorism, Pulmonary stenosis, Abnormalities of genitalia, Retardation of growth, and Deafness, sensorineural (Gorlin et al., 1969). The predominating cardiovascular abnormality is cardiomyopathy—to the extent that an alternative designation is obstructive cardiomyopathy and lentiginosis. There appears to be a great deal of phenotypic overlap with a number of other syndromes including neurofibromatosis, Noonan, Aarskog, and Forney syndromes.

Marfan Syndrome

Marfan syndrome is one of the more readily recognized autosomal dominant diseases and has a prevalence of about 1 : 60,000. The three major areas involved are the eye, the skeleton, and the cardiovascular systems (McKusick, 1972; Pyretz and McKusick, 1979). Affected individuals (Fig. 6-4) are generally taller than their unaffected sibs and have long, thin

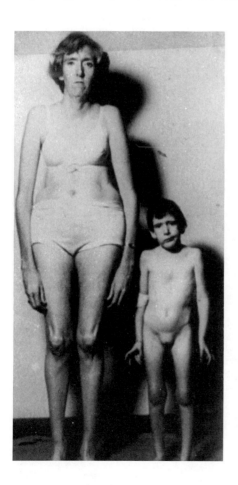

Figure 6-4 Note characteristic phenotypic findings of Marfan syndrome in this mother and daughter.

extremities. The ratios of the upper to lower segments, hand to height, and foot to height offer objective measurements. Kyphoscoliosis, pectus excavatum (or carinatum), and joint laxity are characteristic skeletal abnormalities. Superior temporal subluxation of the lens, iridokinesis, myopia, spontaneous retinal detachment, and blue sclera are common eye findings.

Life expectancy in this syndrome is 32 ± 16.4 years and cardiovascular (CV) disease is responsible for all but a small percentage of deaths; in one series it was the cause of 52 of 56 deaths (Murdock et al., 1972). In another series, CV disease was found in 61% of patients (Phornphutkul et al., 1973), and we estimate from our series studying family members by echocardiography that cardiovascular abnormalities are present in greater than 80% of individuals in whom we make a diagnosis of Marfan syndrome.

The most frequent CV problem is mitral dysfunction, which may be as mild as an apical click with minimal prolapse of the posterior mitral leaflet on echocardiography, or as severe as a ruptured chordae and sudden collapse and death. We have followed patients by echocardiography who have progressed rapidly from mild mitral regurgitation without auscultatory abnormalities to severe mitral regurgitation with florid congestive heart failure, the latter resulting from the distortion and separation of the mitral leaflets progressing in response to the stretching of their supporting structures.

Aortic dilatation with aortic insufficiency and dissecting aortic aneurysm (Fig. 6-5) is the other common CV complication, and is more often implicated than mitral disease in catastrophic episodes leading to sudden death. Ruptured sinus of Valsalva, pulmonary artery dilatation, and an occasional "garden variety" malformation, such as atrial septal defect are also found.

There is an apparent clustering within families of a given type of cardiovascular anomaly. Most often an individual patient and his close relatives will have mitral disease alone. The next most common situation is for the members of a family to have combined mitral and aortic disease. Least common is for a patient to have aortic disease alone and a first-degree relative to have mitral disease alone.

We are convinced that patients with Marfan syndrome must be monitored carefully by echocardiography for evidence of progression of their CV disease. Dimensions of the aortic root, left atrium and left ventricle, as well as mitral valve movements should be followed as a guide to medical management (e.g., when using propranolol), or to anticipate the need for surgical intervention.

Mitral Valve Prolapse (Click-Murmur) Abnormality

The appreciation of mitral valve prolapse through auscultatory findings of an apical mid to late systolic click with or without a late systolic murmur has accelerated during the past decade because of echocardiography (Figs. 6-6, 6-7). Initially there was great concern about this disorder because of

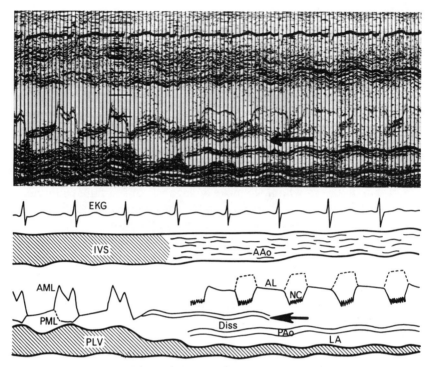

Figure 6-5   Dissecting aneurysm (arrows) of aorta demonstrated by M-mode echocardiography in patient with Marfan syndrome.

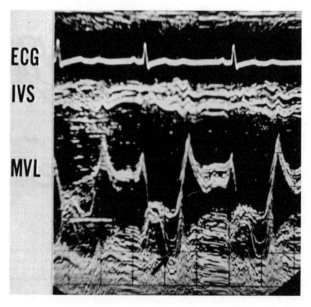

Figure 6-6   Severe prolapse and invagination (arrows) of posterior leaflet of mitral valve.

reports of associated dysrhythmias, sudden death, and subacute bacterial endocarditis (SBE) (Barlow and Bosman, 1966; Stannard et al., 1967; Shappell, et al., 1973). These potentially disastrous consequences of mitral dysfunction led cardiologists to study individuals and families to institute programs of prophylaxis. In a relatively short period of time we accumulated many hundreds of these patients, occasionally with more than one affected first-degree relative, but none with a positive family history of arrhythmia, sudden death, or SBE. Mitral valve prolapse is also found in various connective tissue disorders.

It is now apparent that mitral valve prolapse, occurring in 4–7% of the general population (Devereux and Brown, 1983), is common, heterogeneous, usually sporadic, and that serious complications are uncommon in those without leaflet thickening. Because many cases (particularly the more severe ones) are familial, the condition is discussed in this section. We counsel recurrence risks based on the experience within a given family. For the present we record this disorder as following an autosomal dominant mode in *some* families. The higher-risk patient for infectious and hemodynamic complications has leaflet thickening and redundancy on echocardiographic assessment (Marks et al., 1989).

Our current policy, which may be modified at any time, is to advocate prophylaxis for SBE for those who have leaflet thickening and redundancy, a murmur as well as a click, and not to recommend it for patients who have only clicks. (We are aware that endocarditis has been seen in the

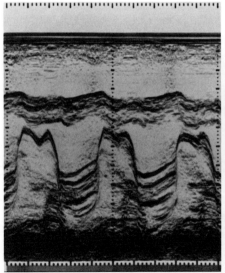
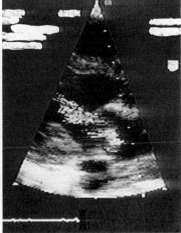

Figure 6-7 Prolapse and redundancy of posterior leaflet of the mitral valve shown in M-mode. The 2-D color flow imaging (in economical black and white) on the right shows the accompanying mitral regurgitation.

"absence" of valvular incompetence, but we feel that the risk of SBE should predictably be greater during regurgitation.) We do not use prophylactic antiarrhythmic agents unless a given patient has an arrhythmia of mainly ventricular origin.

Myotonic Dystrophy (Steinert Disease)

This was the first disease in which autosomal linkage (with secretor and Lewis) was demonstrated. As with so many single-gene disorders, there may be genetic heterogeneity in this condition, which includes among its prominent features the following: myotonia (Fig. 6-8), muscle degeneration, cataracts, gonadal insufficiency, frontal baldness in males, cardiac conduction disturbances, cardiomyopathy, and mitral prolapse. The penetrance of CV disease has been estimated at 65% (most often conduction defects) and there are reports of sudden death, arising presumably from arrhythmias. Hawley et al. (1983) proposed that there may be two forms of myotonic dystrophy based on the tendency to develop conduction disturbances. The evidence is strong for linkage between the loci on chromosome 19 for myotonic dystrophy (DM) and APOC2 (Bird et al., 1987), making it possible in some families that gene probes may be used in prenatal diagnosis.

Neurofibromatosis I (NF I; Von Recklinghausen Disease)

Café-au-lait spots and fibromatous tumors of the skin (Fig. 6-9) are the most common features of this syndrome and may also manifest neural tumors and neoplasms in many other areas. The cardiovascular involve-

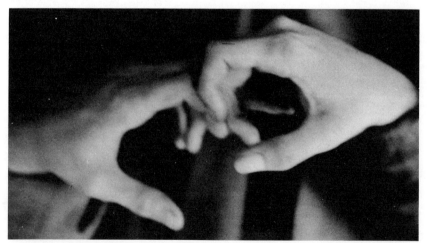

Figure 6-8 Patients with myotonic dystrophy (Steinert) have difficulty in relaxing contracted muscles.

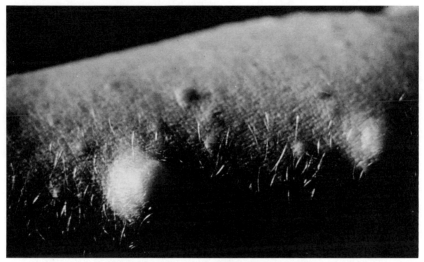

Figure 6-9 Typical neurofibroma (arm).

ment includes hypertension (pheochromocytoma, coarctation of the aorta, renal artery stenosis), pulmonary stenosis (most often valvular), and supravalvular aortic stenosis. From various sources, we estimate the risk of all CV diseases in this syndrome to be 5–10%. The NF I gene maps in the centromeric region of chromosome 17 (Barker et al., 1987).

Noonan Syndrome (Ullrich-Noonan Syndrome, Turner Phenotype)

This syndrome, which has clinical features similar to Turner syndrome, will receive a somewhat longer discussion than the others in this chapter for several reasons. The first relates to how common the condition is, since our estimates place it as the most common autosomal dominant syndrome in our experience. Because half of the patients have cardiovascular malformations (Nora et al., 1974), it is also the most common mendelian cause for congenital heart disease in our clinic. The second reason for a longer discussion relates to diagnostic problems, although this syndrome was fairly well described six decades ago by Ullrich (1930).

This leads to the third reason for an amplified discussion of this syndrome—what to name it—because the syndrome appears in the literature under a variety of names, depending on personal preferences. We will follow what is becoming the convention in the United States by using the term Noonan syndrome. In Europe and other areas, the term Ullrich syndrome has been used for individuals with normal gonadal function who have many of the stigmata we associate with Turner syndrome. We have, in the past, tried to reach a nosological compromise, and have termed the disorder Ullrich-Noonan syndrome to avoid some of the convoluted terminology that was developing (e.g., female-male-Turner). This was not generally adopted. Therefore, we are using Noonan syndrome (for what we have previously called Turner phenotype and Ullrich-Noonan syndrome) to describe those patients, male or female, who have a dominantly inherited disease, normal chromosomes, and certain features (Fig. 6-10) including, in descending order of frequency: characteristic facies, short stature, abnormal ears, undescended testes (in 72% of males), eye problems (e.g., ptosis), low posterior hairline, cubitus valgus, CV disorders, webbed neck, and hand abnormalities.

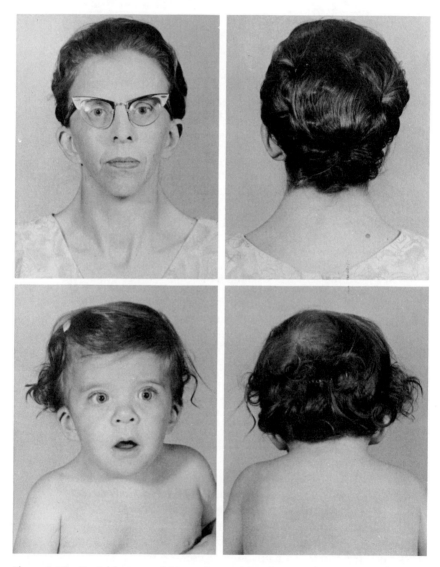

Figure 6-10   Facial features of this mother and daughter are characteristic of Noonan syndrome.

A valuable means of distinguishing Noonan from Turner syndrome on physical examination is to employ the rather sharp dichotomy between their cardiovascular lesions. That is, patients with Turner syndrome have coarctation of the aorta, but rarely have pulmonary stenosis, while patients with Noonan syndrome commonly have pulmonary stenosis, but rarely have coarctation of the aorta.

Another characteristic lesion of Noonan syndrome that is almost as common as pulmonary valve stenosis is cardiomyopathy (Nora et al., 1975), one form of which is called eccentric left ventricular hypertrophy. Although the hypertrophy may involve free walls and is not truly asymmetric septal hypertrophy (ASH), there is usually a 1.3 : 1 septal/left ventricular wall ratio. A septal thickness of greater than 150% of normal is substantial diagnostic evidence. These patients usually do not have systolic anterior motion of the mitral valve. Left axis deviation is common, and accelerated conduction abnormalities are occasionally found. The left ventricular disease is usually benign and may only be detectable by echocardiography. However, we have had one death on our series of Noonan patients with left ventricular disease, so we monitor frequently by echocardiography. Those with evidence of left ventricular disease receive an echocardiogram annually; those without are studied every two or three years for echocardiographic evidence of appearance of this abiotrophy. In addition to obstructive cardiomyopathy, a dilated form may occasionally be seen.

The pulmonary valvular stenosis present in Noonan syndrome is often of a dysplastic type and is frequently accompanied by atrial septal defect. Because of the pulmonary valve dysplasia, the surgical repair is often less satisfactory than in patients without the syndrome. The aortic valve is commonly involved and, indeed, all 4 valves may be dysplastic (Simpson et al., 1969) in a particularly lethal condition that has been incompatible with survival beyond the first months of life. (These infants may have little in the way of appreciable murmurs.) Pulmonary artery branch stenosis is one of the more frequently encountered abnormalities. Common anomalies, such as ventricular septal defect and tetralogy of Fallot are found as are less common malformations such as Ebstein anomaly and total anomalous pulmonary venous return.

The penetrance of features of the syndrome sufficient to make a diagnosis appears to be very high, and the penetrance of some form of CV disease is 50%. Most of our patients reveal evidence of direct transmission of some feature of the disorder, but we have some sporadic cases, which are still insufficient in number to propose a mutation rate.

Osler-Weber-Rendu Syndrome (Hemorrhagic Telangiectasia)

Telangiectasia of mucosal surfaces, face, conjunctiva, and fingers with pulmonary arteriovenous fistulae (McCue et al., 1984) constitute the common findings in this syndrome. Bleeding from all sites is a major problem.

Cirrhosis of the liver, pulmonary hypertension, polycythemia, clubbing, and encephalopathy are occasionally seen.

Osteogenesis Imperfecta (OI)

Because the autosomal dominant types of Osteogenesis Imperfecta (OI) are more common, the disease will be discussed in this section. There are at least four types of autosomal dominant OI one of which is a neonatal lethal form. The two recessive types also include a neonatal lethal form, type II, or OI congenita, in which arterial calcification occurs. The classical tetrad of OI is fragile bones (Fig. 6-11), blue sclera, opalescent teeth, and deafness (although two dominant types have normal sclerae—hearing loss and opalescent teeth are variable). The prevalence of OI is on the order of 1 : 50,000. The molecular defects in collagen in the different forms of OI have been reviewed by Prockop and Kivirikko (1984). As in other connective tissue disorders with CV involvement, mitral valve prolapse, aortic dilatation, and regurgitation are the most common problems (Pyretz, 1983). Although mitral valve prolapse is detectable in 18% of OI type I patients, clinical heart disease is diagnosed in only about 5% of individuals with OI.

Pulmonary Hypertension, Primary

Pulmonary hypertension has important cardiac implications and is a complicating factor in structural malformations of the heart and great vessels. Most patients with pulmonary hypertension do not have the disorder as a primary or isolated condition, but as a complication of cardiac mal-

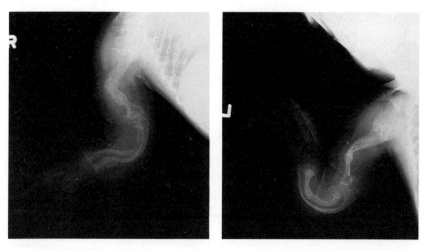

Figure 6-11   Radiographs of multiple fractures in arms of newborn with osteogenesis imperfecta.

development (e.g., ventricular septal defect or transposition of the great arteries). However, there are many documented examples of patients who have pulmonary hypertension as an isolated condition. Some of these cases are familial, conforming to an autosomal dominant mode of inheritance (Melmon and Braunwald, 1963; Parry and Verel, 1966; Loyd et al., 1984). On the other hand, the majority of patients we have seen who have primary pulmonary hypertension do not have an identifiable first-degree relative who has been similarly affected.

Supravalvular Aortic Stenosis With or Without Elfin Facies (Williams-Beuren Syndrome)

The evidence is compelling that this is an autosomal dominant disorder in which different constellations of abnormalities have often diverted attention from a comprehensive view of the syndrome. There are many examples of dominant transmission of supravalvular aortic stenosis (SVAS). Some individuals may have SVAS, supravalvular pulmonary stenosis, or peripheral pulmonary artery stenosis alone or in combination with the other lesions. The familial cases were initially reported to lack the facial stigmata found in Williams syndrome, however, we and others have seen some members of the same family who have SVAS with normal facies, other members with SVAS and elfin facies, and still others with elfin facies and no cardiovascular disease. These families are less common than those without facial abnormalities, but they exist. So do patients with SVAS and normal facies who appear to be sporadic cases.

The role of hypercalcemia and maternal vitamin D exposure must be taken into account. Is there a single-gene abnormality that can be triggered by maternal exposure to vitamin D that leads to a wide range of expression involving, alone or in combination, great vessel disease, smaller artery disease, peculiar facies, hypercalcemia, and mental retardation? A sharp decline in new patients with the syndrome has accompanied the reduced exposure to vitamin D during pregnancy and early infancy in the past two decades.

Our thinking has been influenced by the families we have seen. We puzzled for years over one particular family in which the mother had undeniable elfin facies but no other features of the syndrome. One of her twin children (a boy) had full-blown Williams syndrome, elfin facies, supravalvular aortic and pulmonic stenosis, and mental retardation. His twin sister was normal.

The title of the article from which the eponymic description of Williams syndrome derives is "Supravalvular Aortic Stenosis." (Williams et al., 1961). The possible relationship of the arterial lesion and the peculiar elfin facies to infantile hypercalcemia was suggested two years later (Black and Bonham-Carter, 1963) and was further amplified over the succeeding decade with emphasis on the relationship to vitamin D administration. It has always been the exception rather than the rule, however, to identify elevated levels of serum calcium in a given patient. According to some investigators, the best period to find high serum calcium in these children is between the ages of 4 months and 2 years. The majority of cases, unfortunately, go unrecognized until the patient is beyond 2 years of age. Elevated 1,25-dihydroxy vitamin D levels may be present in the first 2 years of life in the absence of hypercalcemia (Knudtzon et al., 1987).

The "what, me worry?" elfin facies (Fig. 6-12), variable mental retardation, and growth deficiency are associated primarily with SVAS, but valvular, supravalvular, and peripheral pulmonary artery stenoses are also found, as well as occasional septal defects. Beuren (1972) reported a series of 137 patients with SVAS and stressed the familial continuity of the spectrum of elfin facies, mental retardation, and arterial disease. Grimm and Wesselhoeft (1980) have emphasized that this syndrome, now commonly called Williams-Beuren syndrome, is autosomal dominant and may have any or all of the previously mentioned stigmata, including infantile hypercalcemia.

This volume deals with counseling in cardiovascular disease, so our point of reference is the arterial lesion. We do not counsel that these cases are sporadic. Rather, we state that the full syndrome is less likely to recur than only a partial manifestation in the next offspring—for which the risk is

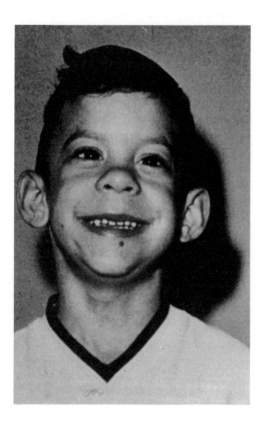

Figure 6-12 Characteristic facies of supravalvular aortic stenosis hypercalcemia syndrome in this boy.

50%. We then stress that the possibility of significant disease may be minimized by protecting future pregnancies and future infants from vitamin D. Our orientation is that the genetic contribution to this disorder may involve only a single locus of "sensitivity" to vitamin D, and that the environmental trigger may be less than the massive doses of the vitamin that produced the epidemic in Germany three decades ago.

Tuberous Sclerosis

This disorder of skin (Fig. 6-13), brain, and bones may also involve the blood vessels, heart, and other internal organs (Lagos and Gomez, 1967). The cardiac disease, most often rhabdomyoma, usually presents as arrhythmias and may be accompanied by electrocardiographic evidence of striking ventricular hypertrophy. Aortic aneurysm has also been described (Larbre et al., 1971). Convulsions or depigmented areas of skin are usually the earliest manifestations. Pitted enamel hypoplasia has recently been recognized as a sentinel finding (Lygidakis and Lindenbaum, 1987). Anticonvulsant and antiarrhythmic therapy are aspects of the medical management. Surgical excision of operable rhabdomyomas may be undertaken. Some tumors shell out smoothly; others cannot be successfully removed. We know of at least one rhabdomyoma that regressed from being "inoperable" at one surgical exploration to being "no longer present" at a later exploration. The penetrance of CV disease (rhabdomyomas and angiomas) is estimated to be moderate.

Velocardiofacial Syndrome

This syndrome (Shprintzen et al., 1981) is characterized by a high frequency of cleft palate, cardiac anomalies, facial dysmorphism, and

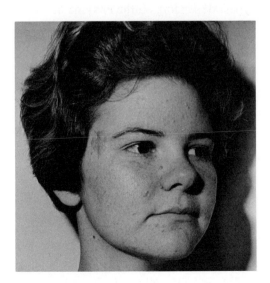

Figure 6-13 Adenoma sebaceum in tuberous sclerosis.

learning disabilities. Also reported are ophthalmologic abnormalities, neonatal hypocalcemia, short stature, microcephaly, mental retardation,
adenoid hypoplasia, frequent infections, and T-lymphocyte dysfunction.
Heart malformations occur in at least half of the patients and are most
often ventricular septal defect and tetralogy of Fallot. The constellation of
abnormalities is what one would see in disruption of the neural crest in
early development.

Von Hippel-Lindau (VHL) Syndrome

Von Hippel-Lindau (VHL) syndrome is characterized by hemangiomas
involving many areas, most commonly the retina and hemangioblastoma
of the cerebellum. Also affected are the lungs, liver, adrenal, face, and
kidneys. Pheochromocytoma produces paroxysmal hypertension which,
when combined with the vascular abnormalites, may lead to cerebral
vascular accidents. Neoplastic changes are not uncommon, especially in
the kidney. The VHL locus maps to the short arm of chromosome 3
(Seizinger et al., 1988).

AUTOSOMAL RECESSIVE CARDIOVASCULAR ABNORMALITIES

Adrenal Hyperplasia

The cardiologist may be the first specialist contacted for this problem,
because of the bizarre electrocardiographic abnormality (see Table 6-2 and
Fig. 6-14) and the circulatory collapse (Sommerville et al., 1968; Nora et
al., 1977). Hyperfunction of the adrenal cortex may be one of several
types, depending on the enzyme involved. About 90% of these cases are
due to a defect of 21-hydroxylase, causing a deficit of hydrocortisone that
stimulates overproduction of pituitary corticotropin. This in turn causes
adrenocortical hyperplasia and excessive androgens and steroid pre-
cursors. The resulting clinical features include virilization of females, but
the male infant may not be recognized until he presents with the CV effects
of hyperkalemia. Potassium retention is associated with sodium loss,
anorexia, dehydration, and vomiting. Myocardial changes, which can be
fatal, are often misdiagnosed as representing structural congenital heart
disease. Potassium retention with its resultant myocardial effects also
occurs in the less common 3-beta-hydroxysteroid dehydrogenase defect.
Virilization is incomplete in these children because androgenic hormones
are not synthesized. Penetrance of hyperkalemia with electrocardiographic and myocardial involvement is almost complete ($\approx$100%) if there is
not prompt recognition and proper treatment. The 21-hydroxylase gene is
located on the short arm of chromosome 6 in the major histocompatibility
complex (MHC). This makes prenatal diagnosis possible through HLA
haplotypes and gene probes (White et al., 1987). The value of prenatal

Table 6-2   Selected autosomal recessive cardiovascular abnormalities

Abnormality	Types of cardiovascular disease
Adrenal hyperplasia	Hyperkalemia, broad QRS, arrhythmias
Alkaptonuria	Aortic and mitral disease, premature arteriosclerosis
Cutis laxa	Pulmonary hypertension, peripheral pulmonary artery stenosis (PPAS)
Ellis-van Creveld	Atrial septal defect (ASD), most commonly single atrium, other congenital heart lesions
Friedreich's ataxia	Cardiomyopathy and conduction defects
Glycogenosis IIa (Pompe)	Cardiomyopathy
Homocystinuria	Coronary and renal thromboses, hypertension
Jervell and Lange-Nielsen	(see Chapter 9)
Meckel-Gruber	Both complex and simple structural defects
Mucopolysaccharidosis (MPS) IH, IS, IV, VI	Coronary artery and valvular disease
Premature senilities (progeria, Cockayne, Werner)	Atherosclerosis, coronary, cerebral
Pseudoxanthoma elasticum	Generalized vascular disease, coronary insufficiency, mitral insufficiency (MI), hypertension
Refsum	Atrioventricular (AV) conduction defects
Sickle cell disease	Cardiomyopathy, mitral insufficiency (85%)
Thalassemia major	Cardiomyopathy
Thrombocytopenia absent radius (TAR)	ASD, tetralogy, dextrocardia

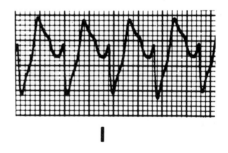

I

II

Figure 6-14 Broad QRS complexes and bradycardia in patient with hyperkalemia and adrenogenital syndrome.

treatment by administering glucocorticoids to the mother has been debated and may reasonably be considered (Pang, 1990).

Alkaptonuria

This is, of course, one of the first 4 mendelian conditions of man, as proposed by Garrod (1902). That there would be a basic defect in the activity of an enzyme was also predicted by Garrod. The features of the disorder are an absence of homogentisic acid oxidase which permits large quantities of homogentisic acid to be excreted in the urine. The urine of affected patients turns black on standing. The absence of the enzyme in the cartilage is responsible for the bluish-black discoloration of the ears and nose. Arthritis occurs in about half of the patients from degeneration of pigmented cartilage. The associated cardiovascular problems are aortic and mitral disease (valvulitis, calcification), and early onset of coronary heart disease associated with generalized arteriosclerosis. Myocardial infarction is a common cause of death. The occurrence of some form of CV disease is considered to be moderate to high (La Du, 1978).

Cutis Laxa

Familial cases of this disorder conform to recessive (three forms), dominant, and X-linked modes of inheritance, with recessive type I being more malignant in terms of cardiovascular-pulmonary involvement (Hajjar and Joyner, 1968). Loose folds of skin and "bloodhound" facies characterize the external appearance of these patients. The internal manifestations of interest include arterial aneurysms, gastrointestinal and genitourinary prolapses and herniation, airway and pulmonary problems producing cor pulmonale, and pulmonary valve and peripheral pulmonary artery stenosis.

Ellis-Van Creveld Syndrome

Chondroectodermal dysplasia is an alternative term for this syndrome of short-limbed dwarfism, post-axial polydactyly (Fig. 6-15), characteristic oral and facial features, and dental and cardiac abnormalities (McKusick et al., 1964). The word chondroectodermal, however, does not encompass the important mesodermal dysplasia manifested in cardiac maldevelopment that affects as many as half of the patients with the syndrome. Atrial septal defect (both ostium secundum and ostium primum) and single atrium predominate among the heart defects.

Friedreich's Ataxia

This progressive spinocerebellar degeneration has a high frequency of associated cardiac disease. One half of the patients die in congestive heart

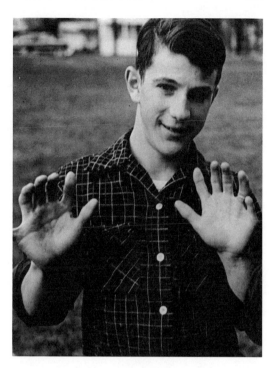

Figure 6-15 Postaxial poly-dactyly in patient with Ellis-van Creveld syndrome.

failure (Hewer, 1968) and 75–90% have some manifestation of CV disease in life—cardiomegaly, S-T and T changes, dysrhythmias, and heart failure.

Glycogenosis II (Pompe Disease)

Glycogenosis II (Ruttenberg et al., 1964; Waaler et al., 1970) is the cardiac form of generalized glycogen storage disease. The deficiency of acid malt-ase produces generalized disease involving the tongue, skeletal muscle, central nervous system, and to a small extent, the liver. Almost all patients have cardiac involvement, although a few exceptional cases have had minimal effects on the heart. Electrocardiographic findings of a short P-R interval and massive ventricular hypertrophy, hypotonia, and an enlarged tongue characterize the clinical presentation. With some exceptions, life expectancy of less than a year is the rule for Pompe (infantile) disease, however, childhood and adult forms are now known (Matsuishi, et al., 1984).

Homocystinuria

There are currently three types of homocystinuria—related to different metabolic defects. Of major interest is the cystathionine beta-synthase (CBS) deficiency, which includes both pyridoxine (vitamin B6) responsive and unresponsive cases. Among its features are inferior subluxation of the ocular lens, skeletal abnormalities that are often similar to those found in Marfan syndrome (Fig. 6-16), malar flush, mental retardation (about one-third have normal intelligence), seizures, psychiatric disorders, and extensive vascular disease. The vascular problems involve thromboses of both arteries and veins and lead to infarction of the myocardium, kidney, brain, and lung. Renal hypertension and gastrointestinal bleeding are other consequences of the vascular disease. This syndrome competes with type IIa homozygous hyperlipoproteinemia as a prominent cause of fatal myocardial infarction in the child. Intimal thickening and deposition of a nonatheromatous ground substance is the histological finding in the vessels of these patients.

Whether the basis for the response to vitamin B6 is allelic or nonallelic has not yet been firmly established. Certainly the progression of the disease in those who are pyridoxine-responsive is impeded by the use of B6. Newborn screening is available so that pyridoxine administration and methionine restriction may be initiated promptly as measures critical to prevention of serious manifestations.

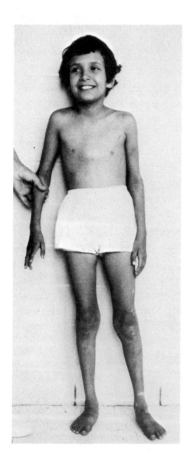

Figure 6-16 Full body view of a child with homocystinuria. The habitus is slim and suggestive of Marfan syndrome. The fingers and toes are not excessively long, nor is the US/LS ratio abnormal.

Heterozygosity for the CBS deficiency is an important risk factor for early-onset occlusive cerebrovascular disease, but perhaps less important for coronary occlusion (Boers et al., 1985). In our experience, even though strokes predominate in heterozygotes, myocardial infarction (MI) is seen in some family members, and both strokes and MIs may occur in the same individual. Testing for heterozygosity by methionine-loading to produce pathological homocystinemia (and by detecting CBS deficiency in cultured fibroblasts) may be useful methods to identify candidates for B6 supplementation and methionine restriction (Mudd et al., 1985) in families ascertained through a homozygote. Such testing may also be considered in families in which there is the unusual family history of strokes and occasional myocardial infarcts in the early decades of life, however, there is concern that the heterozygote may not be reliably detected (McGill et al., 1989). The CBS locus maps at 21q22.3. Brattstrom et al. (1987) reason that if CBS deficiency is in some way involved in the pathophysiology of atherosclerosis, Down syndrome patients might be protected. This appears to be the case.

Hyperhomocystinemia, which may or may not be related to heterozygosity for CBS deficiency, has been emphasized by Malinow (1990) as an independent risk factor for occlusive atherosclerosis including cerebrovascular, peripheral, and coronary artery disease. Treatment of hyperhomocystinemia with pyridoxine and folates has been recommended.

Meckel-Gruber Syndrome

Multiple anomalies of many systems characterize this syndrome (Opitz and Howe, 1969). Encephalocele, polycystic or hypoplastic kidneys, polydactyly, cleft palate, and incomplete genital development are most commonly found. Congenital heart disease, often of a complex and life threatening type, is recognized in as many as 25% of the patients. Simpler lesions, such as ventricular or atrial septal defects, coarctation of the aorta, and patent ductus arteriosus are also found.

Mucoplysaccharidosis (MPS) I, IV, VI

The number of types and subtypes of Mucoplysaccharidosis (MPS) and their phenotypic differences exceed the limits of this presentation. Coarse facies, skeletal manifestations (Fig. 6-17), limitations of joint movement, and mental retardation, however, characterize most types of MPS (McKusick, 1972). Cardiovascular disease is also an important feature, but is notably absent in MPS III. All of the major types are autosomal recessive except MPS II (Hunter syndrome), which is X-linked. Valvular and coronary artery disease progress and contribute to the early death of the majority of affected individuals. The valve most frequently involved is the aortic (regurgitation and stenosis), but all 4 valves may be thickened by

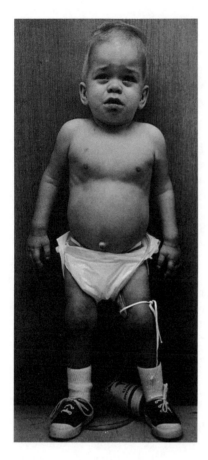

Figure 6-17 Facies in Hurler syndrome
(mucopolysaccharidosis I).

deposition of mucopolysaccharides in a particularly lethal situation which
usually leads to death in early infancy.

Premature Senilities

Progeria

Progeria (DeBusk, 1972) is the most fulminant of the premature senilities
with death occuring as early as 7 years of age. Severe growth retardation,
normal intelligence, loss of subcutaneous fat, alopecia, skeletal hypoplasia
and degeneration, and generalized atherosclerosis characterize the clinical
picture (see Fig. 6-18). Coronary occlusions are more common than cerebrovascular occlusions, and it is these two forms of vascular pathology
that are usually responsible for the early death of patients with progeria.

Cockayne Syndrome

Cockayne syndrome is characterized by growth failure, deafness, retinal
degeneration, mental retardation, unsteady gait, marble epiphyses, dermal
photosensitivity, and premature atherosclerosis. It falls between progeria

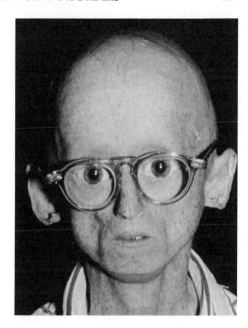

Figure 6-18 Appearance of advanced age in 15-year-old child with progeria.

and Werner syndrome in the speed of its progression to early death. Hypertension is also a common feature. Prenatal diagnosis using sensitivity of cultured cells to UV irradiation has been achieved (Lehmann et al., 1985).

Werner Syndrome

Werner syndrome is not as rapidly progressive as progeria and Cockayne syndrome. The aged facial appearance, early onset of gray hair and baldness, scleroderma-like changes in the skin, cataracts, and diabetes mellitus ($\approx 50\%$) contribute to the picture of premature aging (Fleischmeyer and Nedwick, 1973). Arterial calcification, subcutaneous atrophy and calcification with development of ulcers over bony prominences, organic brain syndrome, and early onset coronary heart disease are other characteristics. The coronary artery disease is more consistent with Mönckeberg calcific arteriosclerosis than atherosclerosis. Aortic stenosis has also been observed.

Pseudoxanthoma Elasticum

Genetic heterogeneity clearly exists (Pope, 1975). However, autosomal recessive is the mode of inheritance in most families having this syndrome of highly characteristic skin lesions, angioid streaks in the ocular fundus, and CV disease. Vascular disease is progressive, and eventually all patients (except the rare families with type II disease) will have generalized calcific arteriosclerotic changes. Death attributable to disease of coronary, cerebral, or renal arteries is customary. Valvular disease, most often mitral or aortic, is becoming more widely recognized because echocardiography is being used to study these families. Systemic hypertension is frequently found as a result of the vascular disease.

Refsum Syndrome

This syndrome has the cardinal features of cerebellar signs, polyneuritis, retinitis pigmentosa, and cardiac conduction defects (Refsum, 1952). Most patients have, at least, an electrocardiographic abnormality. Atrioventricular conduction may be disrupted to the point of complete heart block, requiring pacemaker implantation.

Sickle Cell Disease

This disorder occurs in individuals of African black ancestry. The common cardiac involvement in sickle cell disease is not congenital, but is a progressive disorder with several manifestations related to anemia and iron depositions in the myocardium, cardiomegaly, diminished myocardial function, mitral insufficiency, and occasionally pericarditis (Engle, 1964). The longer the patient survives, the more likely it is that cardiac findings will become apparent. As high as 85% of patients with the homozygous disease have cardiomegaly on x-ray or have electrocardiographic abnormalities. Right-sided heart disease produced by pulmonary hypertension secondary to thromboembolic events may also be encountered. Prenatal diagnosis using DNA polymorphisms is available (Orkin, 1984).

Thalassemia Major

There is progressive cardiac involvement in those who have the severe type of thalassemia major. Myocardial disease and mitral insufficiency are similar to that found in sickle cell disease. In both diseases anemia and iron deposition in the myocardium and papillary muscles appear to be involved. Pericarditis is common, self-limiting, and relatively benign. Cardiac conduction abnormalities are frequently found. In 80% of children who reach the second decade, some form of cardiac complication exists, and in a large proportion of these the complication is a serious one. Prenatal diagnosis (Orkin, 1984) is available as it is for sickle cell disease.

Thrombocytopenia Absent Radius (TAR) Syndrome

In this syndrome (Hall, 1987) of skeletal and hematologic abnormalities, there is a relatively high frequency (20%) of congenital heart diseases. Atrial septal defect, tetralogy of Fallot, and dextrocardia have been reported. The genetics of this problem is not entirely resolved, but that there is an instance of parent-to-child transmission.

X-LINKED CARDIOVASCULAR ABNORMALITIES

Angiokeratoma, Diffuse (Fabry Disease)

Although it is the vascular skin lesions that provide the basis for the name of the disease, the lipid vascular lesions and lipid accumulations elsewhere are the ones of major clinical concern, particularly those in the kidney and heart (Becker et al., 1975). The usual cause of death is renal failure. The vessels of the ocular fundus are prominently involved. Episodic pain in the hands, feet, and abdomen (often misdiagnosed as appendicitis) is a presenting symptom. The metabolic defect is a deficiency of lysosomal alpha-galactosidase A, which permits glycosphingolipids to accumulate in most body cells, including ganglion cells (responsible for the pain), blood vessels, and the heart (myocardial and valvular disease results) (see Table 6-3). Congestive heart failure and stroke are frequently encountered. Intermediate levels of the deficient enzyme and corneal opacities may serve to identify the female carrier. Three DNA markers locate the gene at Xq22 (MacDermot et al., 1987).

Incontinentia Pigmenti

This syndrome is apparently X-linked dominant and lethal in the male. A characteristic "marble cake" skin lesion is associated with malformations of the skeleton, teeth, eye, and heart. The heart lesions include patent ductus arteriosus and cor pulmonale secondary to primary pulmonary hypertension. The IP gene is most likely located in band Xp11.2 (Cannizzaro and Hecht, 1987).

Mucopolysaccharidosis II (Hunter Syndrome)

As in the autosomal recessive mucopolysaccharidoses, coronary artery and valvular diseases eventually become prominent in this syndrome of characteristic facial, skeletal, and visceral abnormalities—without corneal clouding. The manifestations are not as severe as those found in Hurler syndrome (Fig. 6-19), and indeed, there appear to be two allelic forms, a more severe (type A) and a mild (type B). Survival in the severe type A is

Table 6-3 Selected X-linked syndromes with associated cardiovascular abnormalities

Abnormality	Types of cardiovascular disease
Angiokeratoma (Fabry)	Vascular, myocardial
Incontinentia pigmentia X-D	PDA, primary pulmonary hypertension
MPS II (Hunter)	Coronary artery disease, valvular disease
Muscular dystrophy (Duchenne, Becker, and Dreifuss types)	Cardiomyopathy

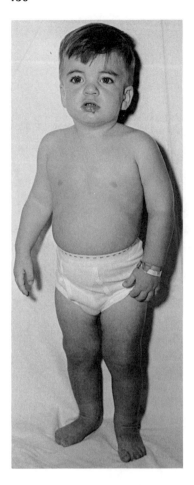

Figure 6-19 Child with Hunter syndrome. Note the facies and the "claw hand."

seldom past the second decade, whereas there are patients with the mild type B who reach the sixth decade. The risk of CV involvement is present in almost all patients. A number of methods for carrier detection have been developed. The Hunter gene is mapped at Xq28 (Roberts et al., 1987).

Muscular Dystrophy (Duchenne, Becker, and Dreifuss Types)

Once could devote many pages to the recent exciting advances in our understanding of muscular dystrophy, but we will avoid the temptation and focus mainly on the CV aspects. In the severe pseudohypertrophic progressive type (Duchenne or DMD), the onset of enlarged calves and muscle weakness is usually apparent by age 6 years (Fig. 6-20) and death usually supervenes before age 20. The Becker form (BMD) has pseudohypertrophy, but is milder. The tardive type of Dreifuss is as early in onset as BMD, but the progress of the disease is slower and characterized by

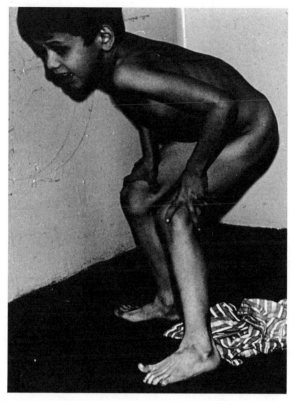

Figure 6-20　Patient with Duchenne muscular dystrophy "climbing up himself."

contractures and a rigid spine (usually in the absence of pseudohypertrophy). Cardiomyopathy and conduction disturbances occur in essentially all cases of DMD, Dreifuss, and often in BMD (but rarely in the autosomal forms). Electrocardiographic changes are early findings (Skyring and McKusick, 1961). Both the Duchenne and Becker types are the result of mutations in the huge gene that encodes for dystrophin (Monaco and Kunkel, 1987). Carrier testing has been possible since the 1970s, but the addition of DNA sequence analysis has revolutionized the approach to DMD, defined numerous deletions, and made prenatal diagnosis a valid clinical option. The extremely large gene has been assigned to Xp21.2 and the cDNA has been cloned (Koenig et al., 1987).

OTHER ABNORMALITIES AND SYNDROMES

Cardiovascular disease has been reported in many other mendelian conditions. Categories such as connective tissue, storage, metabolic, and neuromuscular disorders all have examples of associated involvement of the CV system that will not be represented in these pages. Our selection of conditions for very brief discussion in Chapter 6 may be deemed arbitrary—more accurately, it simply reflects our own experience. Also, there exist a great many syndromes and conditions of CV interest, the formal genetics of which are not clear to us. Chapter 7 is devoted to some of these.

REFERENCES

Barker, D. et al. (1987). *Science*. **236,** 1100.

Barlow, J.B., and Bosman, C.K. (1966). *Am. Heart J*. **71,** 166.

Becker, A.E., Schoorl, R., Balk, A.G., and vanderHeide, R.M. (1975). *Am. J. Cardiol*. **36,** 829.

Beuren, A.J. (1972). In: *Clinical Delineation of Birth Defects*. XV, Williams & Wilkins, Baltimore. pp. 45–56.

Bird, T.D., Boehnke, M., Schellenberg, G.D., Deeb, S.S., and Lipe, H.P. (1987). *Arch. Neurol*. **44,** 273.

Black, J.A., and Bonham-Carter, R.E. (1963). *Lancet* **2,** 745.

Boers, G.H.J. et al. (1985). *N. Engl. J Med*. **313,** 709.

Brattstrom, L., Englund, E., and Brun, A. (1987). *Lancet* **1,** 391.

Cannizzaro, L.A., and Hecht, F. (1987). *Clin. Genet*. **32,** 66.

Cayler, C.G. (1969). *Arch. Dis. Child*. **44,** 69.

Cohen, M.M. (1972). In: *Clinical Delineation of Birth Defects*. XV, Williams & Wilkins, Baltimore. pp. 132–133.

DeBusk, F.L. (1972). *J. Pediatr*. **80,** 697.

Devereux, R.B., and Brown, W.T. (1983). *Progress in Medical Genetics*. V, 139.

Engle, M.A. (1964). *Ann. NY. Acad. Sci*. **119,** 694.

Fleischmeyer, R., and Nedwich, A. (1973). *Am. J. Med*. **54,** 111.

Gall, J.C., Stern, A.M., and Cohen, M.M. (1966). *Am. J. Hum. Genet*. **18,** 187.

Garrod, A.E. (1902). *Lancet* **2,** 1616.

Gorlin, R.J., Anderson, R.C., and Blaw, M.E. (1969). *Am. J. Dis. Child*. **117,** 652.

Grimm, T., and Wesselhoeft, H. (1980). *Z. Kardiol*. **69,** 168.

Hajjar, B.A., and Joyner, E.N. (1968). *J. Pediatr*. **73,** 116.

Hall, J.G. (1987). *J. Med. Genet*. **24,** 79.

Hawley, R.J., Gottdiener, D.S., Gay, J.A., and Engel, W.K. (1983). *Arch. Int. Med*. **143,** 2134.

Hewer, R.L. (1968). *Br. Med. J*. **3,** 649.

Holt, M., and Oram, S. (1960). *Br. Heart J*. **22,** 236.

Knudtzon, J., Aksnes, L., Akslen, L., and Aarskog, D. (1987). *Clin. Genet*. **32,** 369.

Koenig, M., Hoffman, E.P., Bertelson, C.J., Monaco, A.P., Feener, C., and Kunkel, L.M. (1987). *Cell*. **50,** 509.

La Du, B.N. (1978). In: Stanbury, J.B., Wyngaarden, J.B., and Fredrickson, D.S. (eds.). *The Metabolic Basis of Inherited Disease*, ed. 4. McGraw-Hill, New York. pp. 268–282.

Lagos, J.C., and Gomez, M.R. (1967). *Mayo Clin. Proc*. **42,** 26.

Larbre, R., Loire, R., and Guibaud, P. (1971). *Arch. Fr. Pediatr*. **28,** 975.

Lehmann, A.R., Francis A.J., and Gianelli, F. (1985). *Lancet* **1,** 486.

Loyd, J.E., Primm, R.K., and Newman, J.H. (1984). *Am. Rev. Respir. Dis.* **121,** 194.

Lygidakis, M.A., and Lindenbaum, R.H. (1987). *Clin. Genet.* **32,** 216.

MacDermot, K.D., Morgan, S.H., Cheshire, J.K., and Wilson, T.M. (1987). *Hum. Genet.* **77,** 263.

Malinow, M.R. (1990). *Circulation.* **81,** 2004.

Marks, A.R. et al. (1989). *N. Engl. J. Med.* **320,** 1031.

Matsuishi, T., Yoshino, M., Terasawa, K., and Nonaka, I. (1984). *Arch. Neurol.* **41,** 47.

McCue, C.M., Hartenberg, M., and Nance, W.E. (1984). *Am. J. Med. Genet.* **19,** 19.

McGill, J.J., Mettler, G., Rosenblatt, G.S., and Scriver, C.R. (1989). *Am. J. Hum. Genet.* (suppl.) **45,** A54.

McKusick, V.A. (1972). *Heritable Disorders of Connective Tissue,* ed. 4. Mosby, St. Louis.

McKusick, V.A., Egeland, J.A., and Eldridge, T. (1964). *Johns Hopkins Med. J.* **115,** 306.

Monaco, A.P., and Kunkel, L.M. (1987). *Trends Genet.* **3,** 33.

Melmon, K.L., and Braunwald, E. (1963). *N. Engl. J. Med.* **269,** 770.

Mudd, S.H. et al. (1985). *Am. J. Hum. Genet.* **37,** 1.

Murdock, J.L., Walker, B.A., and Halpern, B.L. (1972). *N. Engl. J. Med.* **286,** 804.

Nelson, K.B., and Eng, G.D. (1972). *J. Pediatr.* **81,** 16.

Nora, J.J., Lortscher, R.H., and Spangler, R.D. (1975). *Am. J. Dis. Child.* **129,** 1417.

Nora, J.J., McGrath, R.L., and Wolfe, R.R. (1977). *Chest.* **71,** 686.

Nora, J.J., Nora, A.H., and Sinha, A.K. (1974). *Am. J. Dis. Child.* **127,** 48.

Opitz, J.M., and Howe, J.J. (1969). In: *Clinical Delineation of Birth Defects.* II, Williams & Wilkins, Baltimore. pp. 167–179.

Orkin, S.H. (1984). *Blood.* **63,** 249.

Pang, S. (1990). *N. Engl. J. Med.* **322,** 111.

Parry, W.R., and Verel, D. (1966). *Br. Heart J.* **28,** 193.

Phornphutkul, C., Rosenthal, A., and Nadas, A.S., (1973). *Circulation.* **47,** 587.

Pope, F.M. (1975). *Br. J. Dermatol.* **92,** 493.

Prockop, D.J., and Kivirikko, K.I. (1984). *N. Engl. J. Med.* **311,** 376.

Pyretz, R.E. (1983). *Prog. Med. Genet.* **V,** 191.

Pyretz, R.E., and McKusick, V.M. (1979). *N. Engl. J. Med.* **300,** 772.

Refsum, S. (1952). *J. Nerv. Ment. Dis.* **116,** 1046.

Roberts, S.H., Upadhyaya, M., Sarfarazi, M., and Harper, P.S. (1987). *Cytogenet. Cell Genet.* (abstract) HGM9.

Ruttenberg, H.D., Steidl, R.M., and Carey, L.S. (1964). *Am. Heart J.* **67,** 469.

Seizinger, B.R. et al. (1988). *Nature.* **332,** 268.

Shappell, S.D., Marshall, C.E., and Brown, R.E. (1973). *Circulation.* **48,** 1128.

Shprintzen, R.J., Goldberg, R.B., Young, D., and Wolford, L. (1981). *Pediatrics.* **67,** 167.

Silengo, M.P. et al. (1986). *Clin. Genet.* **30,** 481.

Simpson, J.W., Nora, J.J., Singer, D.B., and McNamara, D.G. (1969). *Am. Heart J.* **77,** 96.

Skyring, A.P., and McKusick, V.A. (1961). *Am. J. Med. Sci.* **242,** 534.

Sommerville, R.J., Nora, J.J., and Clayton, G.W. (1968). *Pediatrics*. **42,** 691.

Spangler, R.D., Nora, J.J., and Lortscher, R.H. (1976). *Chest*. **69,** 72.

Stannard, M., Sloman, J.G., and Hare, W.S.C. (1967). *Br. Med. J.* **3,** 71.

St. John Sutton, M.G., Tajik, A.J., Giuliani, E.R., Gordon, H., and Su, W.P.D. (1981). *Am. J. Cardiol.* **47,** 214.

Ullrich, O. (1930). *Z. Kinderheilk.* **49,** 271.

Waaler, P.E., Garatun-Tjeldsto, O., and Moe, P.J. (1970). *Acta. Paediatr. Scand.* **59,** 529.

White, P.C., New, M.I., and Dupont, B. (1987). *N. Engl. J. Med.* **316,** 1519.

Williams, J.C., Barratt-Boyes, B.G., and Lowe, J.B. (1961). *Circulation*. **24,** 1311.

7

Cardiovascular Disease: Other Syndromes and Disorders

In this chapter we will present a number of conditions in which there is cardiovascular disease—most often as part of a syndrome. All of these disorders have been found to occur in families, but the etiology is unclear in some, while in others different mechanisms appear to have produced the same diagnostic features.

ADDITIONAL MAJOR ANOMALIES

First a note about malformation syndromes. Whatever the cause (major gene, chromosomal aberration, or teratogen), the presence of one major anomaly or three minor anomalies increases the probability that another major anomaly will be found. Cardiovascular maldevelopment is associated with dysmorphology in many systems. If space permitted, complete chapters could be devoted to combinations of heart abnormalities taken one at a time together with each of the following: hearing, skeletal, gastrointestinal, neuromuscular, facial, and renal anomalies.

Sometimes a characteristic combination of anomalies is found in several patients and a syndrome is defined. Major primary malformations involving more than one structure or system may be considered to constitute a syndrome. Many of the conditions that appear in Chapters 6 and 7 could, and probably will be subdivided in the future.

When confronted with a syndrome (a combination of major anomalies involving more than one localized structure), one should suspect a profound genetic (chromosomal or single mutant gene) or teratogenic influence. If the pattern of anomalies does not fit a recognized syndrome of defined etiology, appropriate genetic and teratogenic investigation should be instituted. In this section there are a number of disorders that have been studied (some extensively), but in our view, firm conclusions regarding a single, clear etiology are deficient.

We will not review specific risks of association of one anomaly with another, although there is a small amount of data in this area. The usual counseling situation does not call for answers to questions such as, "given a child with cleft lip and palate, what is the chance that the next child will have cleft lip and palate with cardiovascular disease?'' What is relevant is that, because there is an increased risk of a second major anomaly, one should always be searched for in the patient being examined, even in the absence of precise risk data for various associated problems.

TERATOGEN-INDUCED SYNDROMES

Although the etiologic modes of many of the disorders to be discussed may indeed be heterogeneous, if there is no evidence for a chromosomal or major gene effect, then one may profitably search for a teratogenic influence on simultaneously developing structures and systems.

Examples abound and include the thalidomide, rubella, and fetal alcohol syndromes among others. Sometimes a teratogen may have a very localized effect as with lithium on the tricuspid valve. Other times, several systems or structures may be involved in the absence of a highly characteristic anomaly. VACTERL is an acronym for a condition which simply requires the presence of three or more of the following abnormalities: Vertebral, Anal, Cardiac, Tracheo-Esophageal, Renal, and Limb. VACTERL is not as useful as the thalidomide syndrome with the rare phocomelia as the sentinel deformity. By definition, the thalidomide syndrome and many other teratogen-induced syndromes could be termed VACTERL. And certainly many different teratogens can be implicated in VACTERL, from thalidomide to sex hormones and hydantoin. Perhaps the best way to look at VACTERL is that it reflects an insult to many simultaneously developing structures—this should be the clue to search for a major gene, teratogenic, or chromosomal cause.

Many of the conditions discussed in this chapter (and some in other chapters) may illustrate a mechanism in which the neural crest is disrupted during early development by various means—including teratogens and single mutant genes (see Chapter 4: Pathogenesis). Having reviewed the conditions finally included in this chapter, the authors decided to display a subsection on cardiofacial/neural crest syndromes and to include in Table 7-1 similar syndromes from other chapters (such as the dominant velocardiofacial syndrome). As time passes, several other cardiofacial syndromes may be analyzed from the point of view of neural crest abnormality.

SELECTED DISORDERS

Arteriohepatic Dysplasia (Alagille Syndrome)

The coexistence of biliary dysgenesis (BD), both intrahepatic and extrahepatic, and cardiovascular disease, primarily peripheral pulmonary artery stenosis (PPAS), with or without peculiar facies and other abnormalities, has been recognized for several decades (Sweet, 1932), defined by Alagille

Table 7-1   Other cardiovascular syndromes and disorders

Abnormality	Types of cardiovascular disease
Arteriohepatic dysplasia (Alagille syndrome)	Peripheral pulmonary artery stenosis (PPAS), patent ductus ateriosus (PDA), ventricular septal defect (VSD), pulmonary stenosis (PS)
Atrial myxoma (including Carney)	Intracardiac myxomas, rheumatic heart disease
Cornelia deLange	VSD, TOF, PDA, Double outlet right ventricle
Ivemark	Asplenia with cardiovascular anomalies
Kartagener	Dextrocardia
Kawasaki	Coronary and generalized vasculitis
Klippel-Feil	VSD with pulmonary hypertension, total anomalous pulmonary venous return (TAPVR), transposition of the great arteries (TGA), TOF, ASD, PDA
Rubinstein-Taybi	PDA, ASD, VSD (25%)
Cardiofacial/Neural Crest Syndromes	
Alcohol	(see Chapter 5)
CHARGE	Conotruncal anomalies
Conotruncal anomaly face (CTAF)	Conotruncal anomalies
DiGeorge	Conotruncal, VSD
Goldenhar	TOF, VSD, atrial septal defect (ASD)
Maternal diabetes	(see Chapter 5)
LEOPARD	(see Chapter 6)
Retinoic acid	(see Chapter 5)
Thalidomide	(see Chapter 5)
Velocardiofacial	(see Chapter 6)

et al. (1975), and recently reviewed by Mueller (1987). The introduction of the Kasai operation and the frequency of requests for cardiology consultation from the pediatric surgeons has called our attention to the high frequency of this association.

Heterogeneity definitely exists. LeBreque et al. (1982) has described a four-generation family with Alagille syndrome, which makes autosomal dominant inheritance difficult to deny. A number of other examples of direct transmission are compatible with dominant inheritance. A chromosomal deletion at 20p11.2 has been observed in patients with findings suggestive of Alagille syndrome.

At least two major groups of patients and several subgroups may be derived, taking into account the presence or absence of abnormalities in addition to biliary-hepatic disease and cardiovascular maldevelopment. Half of the patients with intrahepatic ductal hypoplasia in the series of Alagille et al. had a syndrome of characteristic facies, peripheral pulmonary artery stenosis (80%), vertebral anomalies, hypogonadism, growth retardation, and mild to moderate mental retardation (60%). Watson and

Miller (1973) reported a similar syndrome. Many of these patients had associated cardiovascular disease, peculiar facies, and other anomalies. Intrahepatic and extrahepatic BD and neonatal hepatitis also occur with cardiovascular disease without any other stigmata, as well as in a number of other conditions such as rubella syndrome, Zellweger syndrome, and 18 trisomy. About 50% of patients with BD have no significant additional anomalies.

The familial cases of extrahepatic BD have about a 50% risk of cardiovascular disease, and almost half of the patients with intrahepatic BD and PPAS have another cardiovascular lesion, most often pulmonary valvular stenosis, patent ductus arteriosus, or ventricular septal defect. The liver disease in those patients who survive infancy is characterized not only by jaundice and pruritus, but by severe hyperlipidemia and associated stigmata

The etiology of biliary or hepatic disease with cardiovascular disease not related to an established single-gene syndrome (e.g., Zellweger) or chromosomal anomaly (e.g., 18 trisomy) could be teratogenic. The similarity of abnormalities to those in rubella syndrome is readily apparent. Infections and pharmacologic environmental triggers including amphetamines (Levin, 1971) and exogenous sex hormones may be implicated in biliary atresia.

Atrial Myxoma, Familial (Including Carney Syndrome)

Several families in the literature have been recognized who have intracardiac myxomas, most often atrial, but also at other locations within the heart, even in the same family. The inheritance has been compatible with both autosomal dominant and autosomal recessive. A curious relationship exists with rheumatic heart disease in the patient and in first-degree relatives. Bacterial endocarditis is a frequent complication. We have followed a child who had a previous episode of acute rheumatic fever and presented again with apparent rheumatic fever. At the second presentation we discovered a left atrial myxoma by echocardiogram and documented by ultrasound its rapid growth over only a short period of time (Lortscher et al., 1974). An expanded syndrome of familial intracardiac myxoma is the possibly autosomal dominant Carney (LAMB, NAME) syndrome, characterized by the additional features of spotty pigmentation (lentigines) of the skin, subcutaneous neurofibromata, eye abnormalities, and endocrine overactivity—particularly adrenal hyperfunction (Carney et al., 1986).

Cornelia deLange Syndrome

This syndrome (Fig. 7-1) of characteristic facies (with synophrys), limb anomalies, and mental and growth retardation has congenital heart disease as a frequent feature. The heart lesions, present in about 20% of the patients, include ventricular septal defect, double outlet right ventricle,

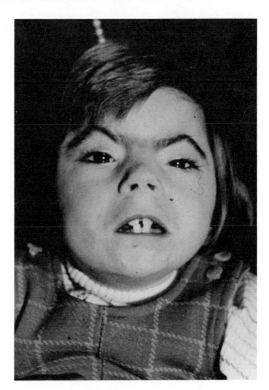

Figure 7-1 Synophrys and thin, down-turned upper lip characteristic of DeLange syndrome.

tetralogy of Fallot, patent ductus arteriosus, and pulmonary stenosis. The chromosomal dup(3q) syndrome has features compatible with deLange syndrome (Wilson et al., 1985). A teratogenic exposure has been detected in some of our cases. Similarities to the Coffin-Siris syndrome have been noted. Autosomal dominant inheritance is favored by some (Bankier et al., 1986) and autosomal recessive inheritance by others (Opitz, 1985). The etiology continues to remain unclear.

Ivemark (Asplenia, Including Polysplenia) Syndrome

Splenic agenesis (or rarely splenic hypoplasia) is often accompanied by symmetric development of normally asymmetric structures and multiple stigmata involving the heart, lungs, abdominal viscera, and red blood cells (Ivemark, 1955). The cardiovascular abnormalities usually include transposition of the great arteries, total anomalous pulmonary venous return, pulmonary outflow obstruction, and endocardial cushion defect. The experience of pediatric cardiologists seeing these patients (and those with polysplenia) reveals that the cases are usually sporadic with a familial recurrence risk on the order of 5%. Three instances of consanguinity in four families of multiply affected sibs in one study (Simpson and Zellweger, 1973), however, provide compelling evidence for single-gene inheritance.

Kartagener Syndrome

Many geneticists, possibly a majority, would list this syndrome of dextrocardia (with abdominal situs inversus), bronchiectasis, sinusitis, immobile cilia, and decreased sperm motility in the autosomal recessive category. Moreno and Murphy (1981) propose that the homozygous state leads to indifferent lateralization during ontogeny. Dominant inheritance has also been suggested. Sinusitis or other features of the disease, alone or in combination, have been accepted as evidence for the presence of the syndrome to meet the 25% expectation required for the syndrome. Sibs of individuals with the full Kartagener syndrome may have coughs, thick nasal secretions, or isolated dextrocardia. Kartagener could represent a subgroup of situs inversus—for which there may be no simple mendelian mode in the human as there is in the mouse (Layton, 1976). Although leaning toward autosomal recessive inheritance, we are still inclined to list Kartagener syndrome in the category of unclear etiology at the time of this writing.

Kawasaki Disease (Mucocutaneous Lymph Node Syndrome)

It is widely assumed that an infectious agent is the triggering factor in this epidemic disorder, which is characterized by a febrile onset with an erythematous rash, conjunctivitis, stomatitis, and lymphadenitis—progressing to a vasculitis (most importantly of the coronary arteries), arterial aneurysms, cardiomegaly, dysrhythmias, and myocardial infarction. Because early diagnosis is valuable in the prompt institution of anti-inflammatory and supportive measures, it is important to recognize that the familial recurrence risk is on the order of 5–10% in siblings (Fujita, 1989), most often in the same time frame, but occasionally months or years later (suggesting a possible genetic predisposition).

Klippel-Feil Syndrome

The core anomaly is fusion and reduction of cervical vertebrae resulting in a short, webbed neck that appears to rest on the chest (Fig. 7-2). A large number of associated anomalies have been described including deafness, neurological impairment, and facial asymmetry. In the past, a treacherous aspect of the syndrome was that the cardiovascular disease often went unnoticed. Having identified a patient with congenital heart disease who had gone undiagnosed, we undertook a study (Nora et al., 1961) of patients carrying the label of Klippel-Feil syndrome (KFS) and found that although over half of them had congenital heart disease, none had been previously recognized as such. The earlier failure to appreciate the high frequency of

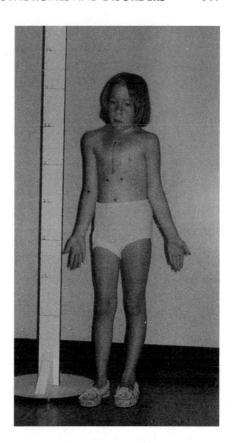

Figure 7-2 Short, webbed neck resulting from fusion of cervical vertebrae characteristic of Klippel-Feil syndrome.

associated cardiovascular disease may have been related to the tendency to focus on the more visible orthopedic and neurologic problems. A more ominous reason is that these patients tend to have rapid development of pulmonary hypertension with associated diminution or obliteration of heart murmurs from left-to-right shunts—thus the consequent failure to recognize the existence of heart disease until it becomes inoperable. We project the risk of heart disease, based on our early series and continuing experience, to be on the order of 25%. If one takes a single cervical vertebral fusion (without reduction in number) as the only diagnostic requirement for KFS, then a case could be made for autosomal dominant inheritance and a lower rate of cardiovascular involvement. Genetic heterogeneity, however, appears to pertain to the expanded syndrome, for which we counsel a low nonmendelian recurrence risk.

Rubinstein-Taybi Syndrome

Broad thumbs and toes, characteristic facies (Fig. 7-3), short stature, and mild to severe mental retardation are prominent features of this syndrome. Recurrence in sibs has been reported, and we have one such family as

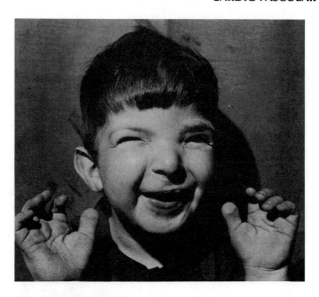

Figure 7-3   Characteristic facial features and broad thumbs of Rubinstein-Taybi syndrome.

patients. Congenital heart disease is present in as high as 25% of the patients and includes pulmonary valvular stenosis, patent ductus arteriosus, atrial septal defect, and ventricular septal defect. Cardiac arrhythmia may follow the use of succinylcholine (Stirt, 1982). The recurrence risk in sibs is on the order of 1%, but the etiology remains obscure. A chromosomal microdeletion has been suggested (Berry, 1987).

CARDIOFACIAL/NEURAL CREST SYNDROMES

CHARGE Syndrome

Coloboma of the eye, Heart anomaly, Atresia (choanal), Retardation, Genital, and Ear abnormalities are the eponymic lesions of the CHARGE syndrome. Choanal atresia is the unusual and life threatening feature (in young infants). Orofacial clefts and abnormalities of the gastrointestinal, genitourinary, and other structures and systems occur (Davenport et al., 1986). About 40% of the cases are familial with both recessive and dominant modes being found (as is the case in multifactorial inheritance). Teratogenic agents have come under scrutiny (Greenberg, 1987). This pattern of anomalies is compatible with disruption of the neural crest in early development. The cardiovascular anomalies are often conotruncal, but ventricular septal defect and atrial septal defect are also seen.

Conotruncal Anomaly Face (CTAF) Syndrome

This syndrome, closely related to the DiGeorge (third and fourth pharyngeal pouch) syndrome, is another example of probable neural crest disruption. All patients studied (Shimizu et al., 1984) had, by definition, conotruncal anomalies (tetralogy of Fallot in 92%). The facies is characterized by ocular hyperteliorism, lateral displacement of the inner canthi, narrow eye fissures, small mouth, flat nasal bridge, and deformed earlobes. The facial features are similar to the velocardiofacial syndrome (see Chapter 6). As compared to DiGeorge syndrome, immune function, the thymus, and parathyroids are less often affected. The authors propose that these patients are on a continuum with full-blown DiGeorge syndrome.

DiGeorge (Third and Fourth Pharyngeal Pouch) Syndrome (DGS)

Anomalous development of derivatives of the third and fourth pharyngeal pouches with neural crest disruption causes a syndrome of aplasia or hypoplasia of the thymus (thymic epithelium) and parathyroids, facial deformities, and anomalies of the heart and great vessels (Freedom et al., 1972). The consequences of the severe cardiovascular disease, (immune deficiency and hypoparathyroidism) usually result in death during the first months of life, however, successful transplantation of the fetal thymus has been accomplished.

In a series of nine patients in Denver who had DiGeorge syndrome (DGS), all had cardiovascular disease, all had ventricular septal defect, and 7 of 9 had additional conotruncal abnormalities (1 truncus, 1 double outlet right ventricle, 5 interrupted aortic arch). Eight of the 9 patients presented as cardiovascular disease and one as pneumonia. We continue to be cautious in our approach to any infant with interrupted aortic arch and are prepared to evaluate for cellular immune deficiency and hypoparathyroidism to avoid undertaking what could prove to be an ill-advised cardiovascular surgical commitment.

Familial recurrences have been compatible with autosomal dominant and recessive inheritance. Partial monosomy of 22pter-22q11 has been seen in both familial and sporadic cases leading some to conclude that a DGS gene could be located in band 22q11 (de la Chapelle, 1981). Teratogenic exposures, including to retinoic acid (Lammer, 1985), have been reported in patients with the features of DGS. The autosomal dominant velocardiofacial syndrome has been proposed to be on a continuum with DGS (Stevens, 1990). It is not unlikely that there are several different causes for the outcome carrying the diagnosis of DiGeorge syndrome.

Goldenhar (Oculoauriculovertebral) Syndrome

The eye, ear, and other facial features of this syndrome are striking, and the epibulbar dermoid is diagnostic (Fig. 7-4). The vertebral anomalies

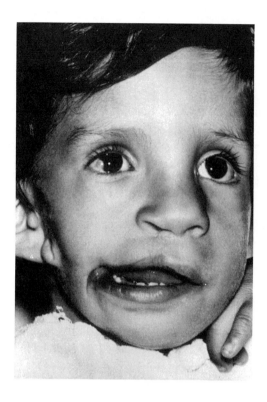

Figure 7-4 Epibulbar dermoid diagnostic of Goldenhar syndrome. Also note cleft lip repair, lateral cleft of the mouth, and ear anomalies.

may be the cause of significant disability, as often as is the associated congenital heart disease. Intelligence does not seem to be impaired. The predominant types of heart defects are tetralogy of Fallot, ventricular septal defect, and atrial septal defect. Our relatively small series shows transposition of the great arteries to be the most common cardiovascular anomaly. The frequency of associated heart disease is as high as 50% (Friedman and Saraclar, 1974; Greenwood et al., 1974). There is evidence for both autosomal dominant and recessive inheritance, and compelling evidence for multifactorial inheritance (Rollnick et al., 1987). The unifying concept here is that Goldenhar syndrome represents yet another example of probable injury to the neural crest.

REFERENCES

Alagille, D., Odievre, M., and Gautier, M. (1975). *J. Pediatr.* **86,** 63.
Bankier, A., Haan, E., and Birrell, R. (1986). *Am. J. Med. Genet.* **25,** 163.
Berry, A.C. (1987). *J. Med. Genet.* **24,** 562.
Carney, J.A., Headington, J.T., and Su, W.P.D. (1986). *Arch. Derm.* **122,** 790.
Davenport, S.L.H., Hefner, M.A., and Mitchell, J.A. (1986). *Clin. Genet.* **29,** 298.
de la Chappelle, A. et al. (1981). *Hum. Genet.* **57,** 253.
Freedom, R.M., Rosen, F.S., and Nadas, A.S. (1972). *Circulation.* **46,** 165.

Friedman, S., and Saraclar, M. (1974). *J. Pediatr.* **85,** 873.

Fujita, Y. (1989). *Pediatrics.* **84,** 666.

Greenberg, F. (1987). *Am. J. Med. Genet.* **28,** 931.

Greenwood, R.D., Rosenthal, A., and Sommer, A. (1974). *J. Pediatr.* **85,** 816.

Ivemark, B.I. (1955). *Acta Pediatr.* (suppl. 104) **44,**1.

Lammer, E.J. et al. (1985). *N. Engl. J. Med.* **313,** 837.

Layton, W.M. Jr. (1976). *J. Heredity.* **67,** 336.

LeBreque, D.R. et al. (1982). *Hepatology.* **2,** 467.

Levin, J.N. (1971). *J. Pediatr.* **79,** 130.

Lortscher, R.H., Toews, W.W., and Nora, J.J. (1974). *Chest.* **66,** 302.

Moreno, A., and Murphy, E.A. (1981). *Am. J. Med. Genet.* **8,** 305.

Mueller, R.F. (1987). *J. Med. Genet.* **24,** 621.

Mueller, R.F. et al. (1984). *Clin. Genet.* **25,** 323.

Nora, J.J., Cohen, M., and Maxwell, G.M. (1961). *Am. J. Dis. Child.* **102,** 858.

Opitz, J.M. (1985). *Am. J. Med. Genet.* **22,** 89.

Rollnick, B.R., Kaye, C.I., Nagatoshi, K., Hauck, W., and Martin, A.O. (1987). *Am. J. Med. Genet.* **26,** 361.

Shimizu, T., Takao, A., Ando, M., and Hirayama, A. (1984). In: *Congenital Heart Disease: Causes and Processes.* Nora, J.J. and Takao, A. (eds.). Futura Publishing Company, Mt. Kisco, New York. pp. 29–42.

Simpson, J. and Zellweger, H. (1973). *J. Med. Genet.* **10,** 303.

Stevens, C.A., Carey, J.C., and Shigeoka, A.O. (1990). *Pediatrics.* **85,** 526.

Stirt, J.A. (1982). *Anesthesiology.* **57,** 429.

Sweet, L.K. (1932). *J. Pediatr.* **1,** 496.

Watson, G.H., and Miller, V. (1973). *Arch. Dis. Child.* **48,** 459.

Wilson, G.N., Dasouki, M., and Barr, M. Jr. (1985). *Am. J. Med. Genet.* **22,** 117.

8

Congenital Heart Disease: Chromosomal Anomalies

When a discovery as important as the method for clinical study of the human chromosome complement became available to investigators, there was a flurry of activity to explore the limits of the new methodology. After some of the common syndromes were defined, it was thought that nonsyndromic, discrete cardiac malformations might also be found in association with gross chromosomal aberrations. This has not so far been the case. While it is unlikely that such an association (in the absence of other abnormalities) will be disclosed, the possibility has not been entirely excluded as high resolution banding techniques are pushed to their limits.

Chromosomal syndromes of small deletions and partial trisomies have proliferated at a rapid rate during the past decade because of banding methodology. Many uncommon syndromes are still inadequately described (from the cardiovascular point of view), and the cardiovascular problems in the common syndromes are so well known that we must reach a compromise concerning the selection of information to be presented. The first point is that, at this stage of our knowledge, when we think of a chromosomal disorder in the etiology of a congenital heart lesion, we should think of a syndrome or multiple system involvement. There should clearly be other manifestations in addition to cardiovascular. If it is a common syndrome, the clinician should recognize it, confirm it by chromosome analysis, and be prepared to find the cardiovascular abnormalities most often reported. If it is uncommon, but the pattern of anomalies leads one to suspect a chromosomal disorder, then, of course, a karyotype will be required. From the point of view of counseling, direct familial transmission of chromosome anomalies producing congenital heart defects (plus other syndromic features) is relatively uncommon. However, heritable translocations and mosaicism will be accompanied by variable increases in familial recurrence risk. It is understood that the counseling must relate to the karyotype, so we will not repeat for each chromosomal anomaly that there is increased risk in the presence of translocation and other abnormalities of chromosome structure and number.

Because familial recurrence is uncommon does not mean that there is no value in clinical genetics to correctly diagnose chromosomal syndromes with associated congenital cardiovascular diseases. The more a physician knows about what his patient has, the more effective will be his management, including that aspect of the art of medicine which Hippocrates called the highest: prognosis. It is also imperative to have a sound clinical and laboratory basis for presenting the best approximation of recurrence risk in the counseling situation.

It is unnecessary to review all catalogued chromosomal aberrations associated with cardiovascular maldevelopment. Table 8-1 displays selected illustrative chromosomal disorders responsible for the majority of cases of such association. The frequency of associated heart disease ranges from as high as 99+% in 18 trisomy to a minimal, if any, increase in structural anomalies in Klinefelter syndrome. The three defects found most often in each syndrome are listed in order, if known. Note that the cardiovascular abnormalities most frequently found in the general population are usually the most common in the autosomal anomalies as well. Coarctation of the aorta, more commonly found in males, predominates in a syndrome which has the absence of an X chromosome (Turner syndrome); patent ductus arteriosus, a malformation more common in females is found when there is an excess of X chromosomes, such as in the XXXXY syndrome.

Table 8-1 Congenital heart defects (CHD) in selected chromosomal aberrations

Population studied	Incidence of CHD (%)	Most common lesions		
		1	2	3
General population	0.6	VSD[i]	PDA[f]	ASD[a]
21 trisomy	40	ECD[e]	VSD	ASD
18 trisomy	99+	VSD	PDA	PS[g]
13 trisomy	90	VSD	PDA	Dex[d]
"22 trisomy" (11 qter trisomy)	67	ASD	VSD	PDA
22 partial tetrasomy (cat-eye)	40	TAPVR[h]	VSD	ASD
4p−	40	ASD	VSD	PDA
5p− (cri-du-chat)	20	VSD	PDA	ASD
8 trisomy (mosaic and partial)	50	VSD	ASD	PDA
13q−	25	VSD	ASD	PDA
18q−	50	VSD	ASD	PS
45,X	20	Coarc[c]	ASD	VSD
XXXXY	24	PDA	ASD	ARCA[b]

[a] ASD = atrial septal defect

[b] ARCA = anomalous right coronary artery

[c] Coarc = coarctation of the aorta

[d] Dex = dextroversion

[e] ECD = endocardial cushion defect

[f] PDA = patent ductus arteriosus

[g] PS = pulmonary stenosis

[h] TAPVR = total anomalous pulmonary valve return

[i] VSD = ventricular septal defect

A detailed discussion of all the clinical features of each of the chromosomal syndromes is not within the purview of this presentation. Instead, we will offer only a brief description of general diagnostic features and a review of the cardiovascular aspects.

AUTOSOMAL ANOMALIES

21 Trisomy (Down Syndrome)

This most common of all autosomal abnormalities has a population frequency of about 1 : 700. Survival is 62% to age 5 and 50% to age 30 in the presence of congenital heart disease. In the absence of heart disease, survival is 87% to age 5 and 80% to age 30 (Baird and Sadevnick, 1987). About 92% of patients with Down syndrome have complete 21 trisomy and about 8% have a translocation or mosaicism. The implications of this in genetic counseling will be discussed later. The general clinical features are summarized in Table 8-2 and are apparent in Figure 8-1. About 40% of patients with Down syndrome have a congenital heart anomaly. Endocardial cushion defect (ECD), most often complete atrioventricular (AV) canal, is followed by ventricular septal defect (VSD) and ostium secundum atrial septal defect (ASD) as the most common heart lesions. (Rowe and Uchida, 1961; Park et al., 1977)

Other common lesions are isolated patent ductus arteriosus (PDA), or

Table 8-2   Features of 21 trisomy

Area	Findings
General	Male sex preponderance (M:F 3:2), variable lengths of survival
Neurologic	Hypotonic, psychomotor retardation
Head	Characteristic facies (patients look more like other patients with 21 trisomy than like their sibs), flat occiput
Eyes	Small, frequently low-set
Nose	Low nasal bridge
Mouth and chin	Protruding fissured tongue secondary to maxillary hypoplasia and narrow palate
Neck	Broad, frequently webbed
Heart	Congenital heart lesions in 40%, endocardial cushion defect most common
Abdomen	Diastasis recti, umbilical hernia, duodenal atresia
Hands	Short hands and fingers, clinodactyly fifth finger
Feet	Gap between first and second toes with plantar furrow
Urogenital	Occasional cryptorchism
X-ray	Pelvic x-rays iliac index < 60°, hypoplasia midphalanx fifth finger
Dermatoglyphics	Simian line, distal axial triradius, ten ulnar loops or radial loops on fourth and fifth fingers
Incidence	1 : 700

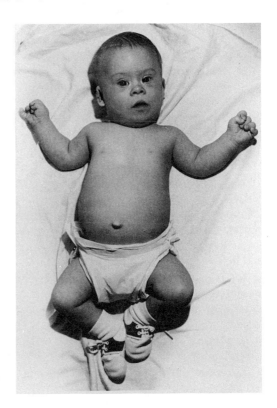

Figure 8-1 Typical appearance of infant with 21 trisomy.

PDA in association with AV canal or VSD, and tetralogy of Fallot. The real discrepancies between the cardiovascular abnormalities in Down syndrome as opposed to those found in the general population are the great overrepresentation of complete and incomplete ECDs and an apparent underrepresentation of transposition of the great vessels.

When following patients with Down syndrome and congenital heart disease, the physician or counselor should be aware of certain special problems. These children have a tendency to develop pulmonary hypertension more rapidly than other children with the same apparent anatomic abnormality. One possible explanation for this is that they do not truly have the same anatomic defect and that an unsuspected PDA contributes high flow under high pressure to the lungs of children who have been followed prior to heart catheterization with only VSD or AV canal. However, there also appears to be a high degree of sensitivity of the pulmonary arterioles of young patients to changes in oxygen concentration. The point is, that if surgery is considered, a much earlier and more aggressive approach in children with Down syndrome may be required.

Another precaution is that what appears to be a straightforward diagnosis often is not. Usually a left-axis deviation on the electrocardiogram will sort out the ECDs from other shunting lesions. But there are many exceptions that can damage the ego of the diagnostician. We have seen ECDs without the sentinel finding of left-axis deviation, and have found patients with ostium secundum ASD, PDA, and VSD (Becu types 2 and 4, as well as 3) who had left-axis deviation.

The first question of the parents, before the questions of etiology and familial recurrence, regards the outlook for and management of the heart disease in their child. This is a very personal and difficult problem. The parents should be full participants in the decision making, and trusted family advisors should be welcome. We have seen families travel halfway around the world with children having Down syndrome, severe heart disease, retardation, and additional handicaps. The trips were made with no guarantee, but with the hope only that heart surgery would be possible. We have seen other families living within a few blocks of the medical center who declined even to have diagnostic cardiac catheterization for their child. In some families the child with Down syndrome is an integral and beloved family member. This is the reason given for desiring surgery or for wishing to avoid the not inconsiderable risk of surgery. In other situations the infant or child has become a burden that threatens to destroy the family unit and surgery is desired or declined in that particular context.

If the heart defect is a simple VSD, ASD, or PDA unaccompanied by severe pulmonary hypertension, the prognosis after surgery can be optimistic for longevity and for the opportunity afforded the patient to achieve maximal physical potential. If the anatomic or physiologic derangement of the heart is more complex, then the prognosis must be more guarded.

No large series is available to contradict the current impression that the type of heart defects and the natural history of these defects are the same in Down syndrome produced by complete 21 trisomy, translocation, or mosaicism. The recurrence risk of a chromosomal anomaly following the birth of an infant with complete 21 trisomy (normal parents) is 1–2%, as it is for other so called sporadic chromosomal aberrations. The risk is less than 5% for recurrence of an unbalanced translocation if the father carries a balanced translocation, but about 10% (depending on the type of translocation) if the mother is a balanced translocation carrier. The risk for familial recurrence in offspring of mothers who have mosaicism in which there is a 47, XX, +21 cell line is increased, but there are insufficient data to define the level of increased risk. We are always wary of the young, not-too-bright mother of a patient with Down syndrome, who might herself have occult mosaicism. When the question arises, a karyotype of the mother is indicated before definitive counseling is given.

Amniocentesis is a preventive measure for mothers over 35 years old, for pregnancies in which there is abnormal maternal serum alpha fetoprotein (AFP), unconjugated estriol (uE3), human chorionic gonadotrophin (hCG), and for families who have had a previous child with a chromosomal abnormality or in which there is a parent with a balanced translocation or mosaicism. It should be noted here that laboratories are far from agreement on the uses and abuses of the newer maternal serum screening methods, and even on the more established maternal serum AFP (Macri et al., 1990).

18 Trisomy

This, the second most common autosomal trisomy syndrome (Taylor, 1968; Hodes et al., 1978; Moerman et al. 1982), has a population frequency rate of 1 : 3,500–1 : 8,000. The clinical features are summarized in Table 8-3 and some are illustrated in Figures 8-2 and 8-3. Congenital heart disease is almost invariably found. We are aware of only one case in which heart disease was reported to be absent. The most common heart lesions are VSD, PDA, ASD, and coarctation of the aorta. Pulmonary stenosis (PS) is frequently found as is polyvalvular disease (Matsuoka et al., 1983). If one looks at a population of patients with 18 trisomy by echocardiography, polyvalvular disease may be the most common cardiovascular problem. It is the rule rather than the exception for an infant with this syndrome to have more than one heart defect (e.g., VSD plus PDA or ASD). Pulmonary hypertension is common. The course of the disease is usually more benign in partial trisomies and mosaics, and the risk of congenital heart disease appears to be less than in complete 18 trisomy, but the majority of these infants also have heart lesions. Life expectancy in this syndrome is 2–3 months for males and 10 months for females, which introduces a problem

Table 8-3 Features of 18 trisomy

Area	Findings
General	Female sex preponderance (M:F 1:4), low birth weight for gestational age, failure to thrive, early death
Neurologic	Mental and growth retardation, hypertonic
Head	Prominent occiput
Eyes	Epicanthic folds, small palpebral fissures
Ears	Low-set, malformed
Mouth and chin	Micrognathia, narrow palatal arch, microstomia, infrequently cleft lip or palate, or both
Thorax	Short sternum, eventration of diaphragm
Heart	Congenital heart anomalies in 99+%, most often ventricular septal defect or patent ductus arteriosus, polyvalvular disease
Abdomen	Meckel's diverticulum, inguinal hernia
Hands	Third and fourth fingers clenched against palm with second and fifth fingers overlapping them
Feet	Rocker-bottom shape, great toe dorsiflexed
Pelvis	Small pelvis, limited hip abduction
Urogenital	Renal anomalies, cryptorchism
X-ray	Hypoplastic sternum, thin tapered ribs, hypoplastic mandible, "antimongoloid" pelvis
Dermatoglyphics	Characteristic digital pattern of six to ten low arches, high axial triradius, single flexion crease on digits
Incidence	1 : 3,500–1 : 8,000

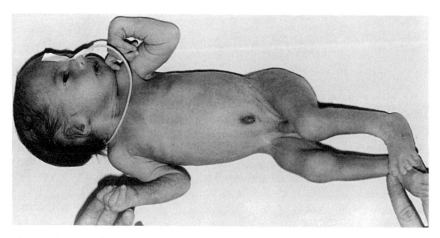

Figure 8-2 Full figure of infant with 18 trisomy showing prominent occiput and overlapping fingers.

regarding the desirable approach to medical management of the patient and the heart disease. Many take the position that cardiac catheterization and aggressive therapy are unjustified.

The counseling in this syndrome is, of course, that the risk of recurrence of complete 18 trisomy in a given family is small. Familial cases of partial trisomies, however, have been reported and the 1–2% risk of some chromosomal anomaly obtains.

Decreased maternal serum AFP is a screening clue to the three most common autosomal trisomy syndromes (21, 18, and 13). Amniocentesis is suggested in cases of abnormal maternal serum AFP, uE3, and hCG, as well as instances where there has been a sibling with a chromosomal anomaly or a parent with a balanced translocation.

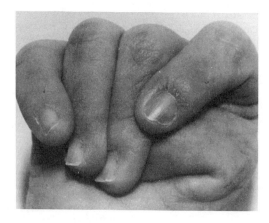

Figure 8-3 Typical overlapping fingers in baby with 18 trisomy.

13 Trisomy

The next most common complete trisomy is of chromosome 13 (Taylor, 1968; Hodes et al., 1978). The population frequency rate is approximately 1 : 4,000–1 : 15,000 and mean life expectancy is 130 days with nearly half dying during the first months. Table 8-4 presents the clinical features and Figure 8-4 illustrates some of these. Congenital heart disease if found in about 90% of infants with this syndrome. VSD, PDA, complex dextroversion, tetralogy of Fallot, and ASDs are the most common abnormalities of the cardiovascular system. As in 18 trisomy, the coexistence of more than one heart lesion is the rule. Complex dextroversion often includes (in some combination), in addition to dextroposition of the heart with normal situs of the abdominal organs, single ventricle, L-transposition of the great arteries, single atrium, total anomalous pulmonary venous return, and pulmonary stenosis. The mirror image of the above may also occur (i.e., normal position of the heart with abdominal situs inversus and cardiac anomalies). How well any of the heart lesions are tolerated depends on the hemodynamic state of cardiac output and oxygenation that is ultimately reached.

The most frequent translocation in the general population is t(DqDq). This occurs in about 1 : 1,000. The majority of individuals having a D/D translocation, most often t(13q14q), are balanced carriers. The risk of a chromosomal anomaly occurring among the offspring of a D/D carrier is reported to be 5% regardless of the sex of the parent. The anomaly is most often an unbalanced D translocation, but may be a complete 21 trisomy. Amniocentesis should be recommended in a family in which one parent

Table 8-4   Features of 13 trisomy

Area	Findings
General	Equal sex distribution, failure to thrive, apneic spells, early death
Neurologic	Mental and motor retardation, hypertonic or hypotonic, defects of the forebrain (holoprosencephaly, arhinencephaly)
Head	Sloping forehead, scalp defects, microcephaly
Eyes	Colobomata, microphthalmia, anophthalmia
Ears	Low-set, malformed
Mouth and chin	Usually cleft lip or palate or both, micrognathia
Heart	Congenital heart lesions in 90%, most often ventricular septal defect, patent ductus arteriosus, and rotational anomalies
Abdomen	Rotational anomalies, hernias, absent spleen, accessory spleens
Hands	Polydactyly, frequently third and fourth fingers clenched against palm with second and fifth fingers overlapping, hyperconvex nails
Feet	Polydactyly, frequently rocker-bottom shape
Urogenital	Polycystic kidneys, hydronephrosis, cryptorchism, bicornuate uterus
Dermatoglyphics	Ridge hypoplasia, radial loops and arches, high triradius, single palmar flexion crease, hallucal arch fibular or fibular-S pattern
Incidence	1 : 4,000–1 : 15,000

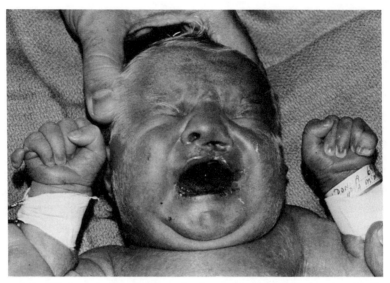

Figure 8-4 13 trisomy with cleft lip and palate, microphthalmia, overlapping fingers and polydactyly.

has a balanced t(DqDq) or if there has been a previous pregnancy with complete trisomy 13. The heart anomalies and severity of the syndrome appear to be the same whether the karyotype is complete trisomy 13 or 13q trisomy. Nonfamilial "phenocopies" with normal chromosomes have also been found and have similar heart lesions. Low levels of serum AFP are found in pregnancies with trisomy 13 and are also an indication for amniocentesis.

We agree with the same restrained diagnostic and therapeutic approach for these patients as for patients with 18 trisomy.

"22 Trisomy" (11qter Trisomy)

This syndrome (Gustavson et al., 1976; Zellweger et al., 1976) is probably not aneuploidy of chromosome 22, but may represent trisomy of 11 qter with a 3 : 1 segregation of the reciprocal translocation. Clinical features are shown in Table 8-5 and Figure 8-5. About 67% of patients with this very rare syndrome appear to have congenital heart disease, usually of the less life threatening varieties. Atrial septal defect is most common, followed by VSD and PDA. Familial recurrence of the syndrome has been repeated in offspring of a mother who had mosaicism involving a "22 trisomy" cell line. The prognosis for longevity is variable and retardation is usually severe. The decision regarding heart surgery is similar to that in Down syndrome. The physician may certainly present the possibility of surgery to the parents, if a low-risk heart operation could make the child more comfortable and make the medical management more effective. The very

Table 8-5 Features of "22 trisomy" (11 qter trisomy)

Area	Findings
General	Equal sex ratio, failure to thrive
Neurological	Mental and growth retardation
Head	Microcephaly
Ears	Low-set, angled, malformed, preauricular tags
Nose	Anteverted nares
Mouth and chin	Cleft palate, micrognathia
Neck	Redundant skin folds
Heart	Anomalies in 67%
Extremities	Abnormal thumbs (digitalized or broad), cubitus valgus, dislocation of the hip
Dermatoglyphics	Excess of whorls, distal axial triradius

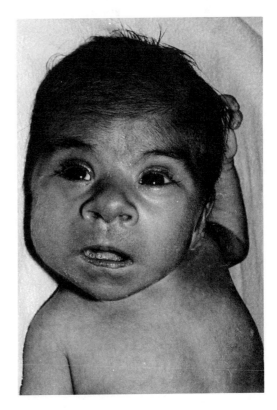

Figure 8-5 Microcephaly, micrognathia, low-set ears, and redundant skin neck folds are common features of "22 trisomy" (11 qter trisomy).

personal decision may be made for or against surgery in the context of fully informed options.

22 Partial Tetrasomy (Cat-Eye Syndrome)

This syndrome (Table 8-6 and Fig. 8-6) is produced by the addition to the normal chromosome complement of a small acrocentric chromosome, which has been confirmed by banding techniques as representing partial tetrasomy 22, a derivative chromosome consisting of a duplication of the centromeric portion 22 pter q11 (Schinzel et al., 1981). There is a 3 : 1 preponderance of females. Coloboma of the iris (cat-eye) and anal atresia are cardinal features. Mental retardation is mild to moderate. About 40% of patients with partial 22 tetrasomy have congenital heart disease, and in the majority of cases it is accompanied by cyanosis. Complex total anomalous pulmonary venous return associated with other abnormalities, such as tricuspid atresia, is the most common defect of the cardiovascular system (Freedom and Gerald, 1973). Ventricular septal defect, ASD, and tetralogy of Fallot are also found. Mosaicism is common in this syndrome, so familial recurrence is a theoretical possibility (which to our knowledge has not yet been reported). Adults without heart disease are now known who have this chromosomal abnormality.

4p Monosomy (4p- Syndrome)

This chromosomal aberration arises de novo in 90% of the cases, but is related to a parental translocation or mosaicism in 10%. Clinical features (Guthrie et al., 1971; Lazjuk et al., 1980) are summarized in Table 8-7 and illustrated in Figure 8-7. Congenital heart disease is found in about 40% of the patients. The number of patients is still so few that the frequency rate of congenital heart disease can change as new cases are reported. It is perhaps better to bear in mind that heart disease is not present in the majority of cases. When heart disease actually is present, it is usually one

Table 8-6 Features of cat-eye syndrome

Area	Findings
General	Female sex preponderance (M : F 1 : 3)
Neurological	Mild to severe mental retardation
Eyes	Cat-eye (coloboma of iris), antimongoloid palpebral fissures
Ears	Low-set ears with preauricular sinuses and appendages, deafness
Heart	Heart lesions in 50%, complex life threatening defects, total anomalous pulmonary venous return
Gastrointestinal	Anal atresia
Genitourinary	Renal aplasia
Extremities	Digitalized thumbs, congenital dislocation of the hips

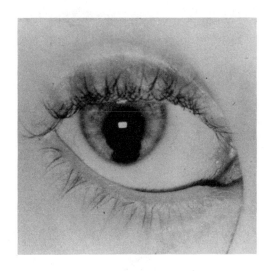

Figure 8-6 Coloboma of the iris is a distinguishing feature of 22 partial trisomy (cat-eye syndrome).

of the common and discrete varieties, such as ASD, VSD, or PDA. Again the risk/benefit ratio should be taken into account before aggressive interventions are undertaken. The risk of familial recurrence can be determined by karyotyping the parents as well as the affected individual.

5p Monosomy, (5p-, Cri-du-chat Syndrome)

This syndrome has physical features (Berg et al., 1970; Niebuhr, 1978) which by themselves are not pathognomic (see Table 8-8 and Fig. 8-8), but has a plaintive, mewing cry that is diagnostic. The frequency of this relatively uncommon disorder is about 1 : 50,000. The loss of a very small segment in the 5p14p15 bands is responsible for the major symptoms. The

Table 8-7 Features of 4p monosomy

Area	Findings
General	Female sex preponderance (M : F 1 : 2), variable length of survival
Neurologic	Mental, motor, and growth retardation, seizures, hypotonic
Head	Microcephaly, prominent glabella, broad nasal root, moon-face, midline scalp defects
Eyes	Colobomata, stasis, nystagmus, strabismus, epicanthus
Ears	Large, floppy, low-set, preaurical tags
Nose	Misshapen
Mouth and chin	High-arched palate, micrognathia, occasional cleft lip or palate or both
Heart	Congenital anomalies in 40%
Extremities	Clubbed feet, deformities of fingers and nails
Dermatoglyphics	Distal axial triradius, low ridge count, frequent arches, hypoplastic dermal ridges

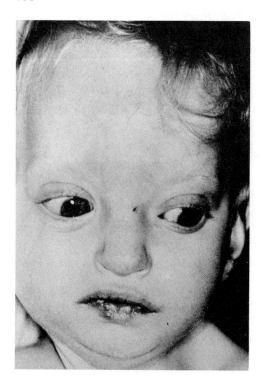

Figure 8-7 Prominent glo-
bella and widely spaced eyes
with inner canthic folds occur
in patients with 4p- syndrome.

deletion is most often a rare sporadic event, however, familial translocations and ring chromosomes are seen often enough to require parental
karyotyping in order to provide optimal genetic counseling. Maternal
transmission is more common than paternal transmission. As cases have
accumulated, it has become apparent that earlier estimates of the frequency rate of congenital heart disease was too high. It appears that only
about 20% have heart anomalies, most commonly VSD, PDA, and ASD.

Table 8-8   Features of cri-du-chat (5p monosomy)

Area	Findings
General	Female sex preponderance (M : F 1 : 2), mewing cry in infancy and early childhood, variable lengths of survival (often to adulthood)
Neurologic	Severe mental retardation, motor and growth retardation
Head	Microcephaly, moon-face, paradoxical alert expression
Eyes	Epicanthus, antimongoloid slant, hypertelorism
Mouth and chin	Retrognathia
Heart	Congenital cardiovascular anomalies in 20%, most often ventricular septal defect or patent ductus arteriosus
Dermatoglyphics	Distal axial triradius (t'), increased whorls, high ridge count
Incidence	1 : 50,000

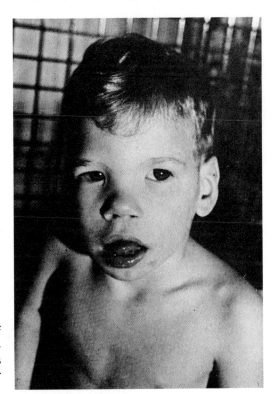

Figure 8-8 Facial features of 5p- syndrome are not pathognomonic. This patient shows wide-spaced eyes with an inner canthic fold.

In the absence of severe congenital heart disease, survival into adulthood is common.

8 Trisomy (Mosaic and Partial)

The majority of cases are mosaic (Fineman et al., 1975; Riccardi, 1977), however, this is one of the two group-C chromosomes in which complete and homogeneous trisomy has been reported (the other is 9 trisomy). Familial recurrence has thus far been confined to partial trisomies. The clinical features are reviewed in Table 8-9. Congenital heart lesions occur in fewer than half the patients and those defects that are common in the general population are the ones most frequently seen. Of particular diagnostic value are the "what-me-worry?" facies (Fig. 8-9) and the deep grooves in the palms and soles of the feet.

Of potential investigative interest in the group-C chromosomes is an observation concerning 9 trisomy. Although complete 9 trisomy, 9q trisomy, and 9p monosomy have risks of associated cardiovascular disease, the most common and recognizable syndrome involving chromosome 9, 9p trisomy, almost never has cardiovascular involvement.

Table 8-9   Features of 8 trisomy

Area	Findings
General	Male sex preponderance (M : F 2 : 1)
Neurological	Mild to moderate retardation
Facies	Prominent lower lip, micrognathia, occasional strabismus, often similar to Williams syndrome
Ears	Large, low-set, sometimes simple
Thorax	Kyphoscoliosis, vertebral anomalies, extra ribs, occasional spina bifida
Heart	< 50% prevalence, discrete lesions (e.g., VSD, ASD, PDA)
Limbs	Ankylosed joints, clubfoot, camptodactyly, clinodactyly, arachnodactyly, brachydactyly, absent patella
Urogenital	Hypogonadism
Dermatoglyphics	Deep grooves (plis capitonnés) on palms and soles

13q- Syndrome

In this deletion syndrome (Allerdice et al., 1969; Niebuhr, 1977), the distinctive physical features (Table 8-10 and Fig. 8-10) are produced by monosomy 13q3. The retinoblastoma gene is found in band 13q14. Approximately 25% of affected individuals have congenital heart disease, the most common heart lesions being VSD, ASD, and PDA.

The 18q- Syndrome (18q2 Monosomy)

The physical features (Wertelecki and Gerald, 1971; Wilson et al., 1979) of the 18q- syndrome are attributable to 18q2 monosomy and are summarized in Table 8-11 and illustrated in Figure 8-11. Heart disease is found in 35% of

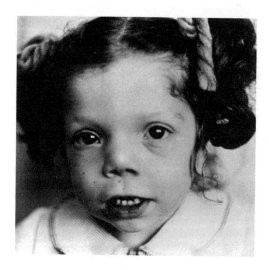

Figure 8-9 The "what-me-worry?" facies reminiscent of Williams syndrome is common in patients with 8 trisomy. This patient has an 8 duplication resulting from an inversion.

Table 8-10   Features of 13q- syndrome

Area	Findings
General	No apparent sex preponderance, variable lengths of survival
Neurologic	Psychomotor retardation, hypotonic
Head	Microcephaly, facial asymmetry, midline facial prominence of glabella with broad nasal root and bridge (trigonocephaly)
Neck	Frequently webbed
Eyes	Hypertelorism, microphthalmus, epicanthus, ptosis, colobomata, retinoblastoma
Ears	Low-set, malformed
Mouth and chin	Micrognathia
Heart	Congenital heart defects in 25%
Hands	Hypoplastic or absent thumbs, short fifth fingers
Urogenital	Hypospadias, cryptorchism
Anus	Occasionally imperforate
Dermatoglyphics	Distal axial triradius (t′), high ridge count with preponderance of whorls, simian lines

patients and usually consists of common lesions such as VSD, ASD, pulmonary stenosis, and PDA.

SEX CHROMOSOMAL ANOMALIES

The 45,X Turner Syndrome

From the cardiovascular point of view, Turner syndrome is the most important of the sex chromosomal anomalies. The clinical features of the

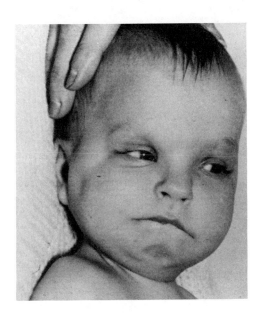

Figure 8-10   Facial features of a patient with 13q- syndrome.

Table 8-11   Features of 18q- syndrome

Area	Findings
General	Equal sex distribution, variable length of survival, low pitched voice
Neurologic	Mental, motor, and growth retardation, hypotonic
Head	Microcephaly, midface hypoplasia
Eyes	Hypertelorism, epicanthus, nystagmus, fundoscopic abnormalities
Ears	Prominence of helix, antihelix or antitragus or both, atretic canals with impaired hearing
Mouth and chin	Downward-turned ''carp mouth'', jutting jaw
Heart	Congenital malformations in 35%
Extremities	Long tapering fusiform fingers, dimpled knuckles, elbows, and knees, club feet, frog position of the legs
Urogenital	Cryptorchism
Dermatoglyphics	High ridge count, preponderance of whorls (> 5)

syndrome (Lemli and Smith, 1963; Rosenfeld and Grumbach, 1989) are reviewed in Table 8-12 and some features are illustrated in Figure 8-12. Approximately 1:2,500 phenotypic females have a 45,X chromosomal constitution. Of these, about 20% have significant hypertension unrelated to coarctation of the aorta. There is such an overlap between the pheno-

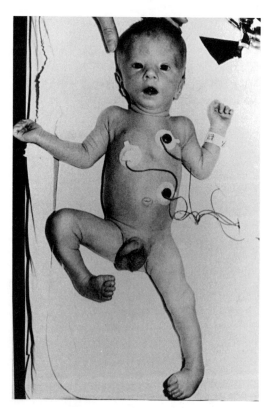

Figure 8-11 Hypertelorism, inner canthic folds, and midface hypoplasia is present in a patient with 18q- syndrome.

Table 8-12 Features of the 45,X Turner syndrome

Area	Findings
General	Sex preponderance (M : F 1 : 2), normal life expectancy may be altered by cardiovascular or renal disease, invariably small stature for age with eventual height attainment rarely exceeding 60 inches, chromatin-negative
Neurologic	Intellectual development is generally good but is usually below the attainment of siblings, perceptive hearing loss is common
Skin	Frequent pigmented nevi
Head	Characteristic facies, narrow maxilla, small mandible
Eyes	Frequent epicanthic folds, occasional ptosis, infrequent hypertelorism
Ears	Usually prominent and low-set
Mouth	Sharklike, curved upper lip, straight lower lip
Neck	Low posterior hairline, webbed in about 50% of patients
Chest	Shield-shaped, widely spaced hypoplastic nipples, underdevelopment of breasts
Cardiovascular	Abnormalities in approximately 20%, coarctation of the aorta is most common, pulmonic stenosis rarely if ever occurs, occasional essential hypertension, bicuspid aortic valve
Extremities	Cubitus valgus, lymphedema of dorsum of hands and feet in infancy, dystrophic nails, short fourth and fifth metacarpals, short fifth finger with clinodactyly, medial tibial exostosis
Urogenital	Ovarian dysgenesis with infertility (only 6 reported instances of fertility)
X-ray	Hypoplasia of lateral ends of clavicles and sacral wings, platyspondylia, metaphyseal dysplasia of long bones, "positive metacarpal sign" (short fourth and fifth metacarpals)
Dermatoglyphics	Distal axial triradius in 20–30%, higher than average ridge count
Incidence	1 : 5,000 (1 : 2,500 females)

types of 45,X Turner syndrome and Noonan syndrome that they are often hard to distinguish in females on the basis of external features. A useful diagnostic dichotomy in the cardiovascular system, however, does exist. If the patient has the coarctation of the aorta, she almost invariably has Turner syndrome; if the patient has pulmonary valve stenosis, she has, with almost no exceptions, Noonan syndrome.

Structural anomalies of the X chromosome associated with Turner syndrome, such as isochromosomes of the long arm, may be accompanied by the same cardiovascular abnormalities as are found in the complete 45,X anomaly. Some X/XX mosaics, however, have been reported to have either pulmonary stenosis or coarctation of the aorta (Nora et al., 1970). An explanation for this could be that those with pulmonary stenosis had a 46,XX constitution (and the dominant gene mutation of Noonan syndrome) up to the point of second cell division, at which time two viable cell lines became established.

Studies of aborted fetuses support the hypothesis that there is a pathogenetic relationship between lymphatic obstruction and cardiovascular

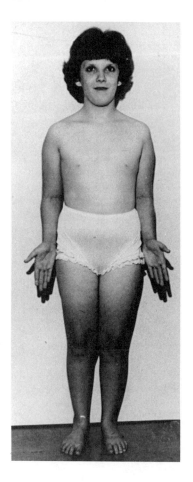

Figure 8-12 Short stature with narrow maxilla, small mandible, shield chest, and lack of secondary sexual characteristics are present in this 14-year-old girl with 45,X Turner syndrome.

maldevelopment in Turner syndrome (Larco et al., 1988). Although co-arctation of the aorta accounts for two-thirds of the cardiovascular disease in these patients, other common malformations occur, such as bicuspid aortic valve (Miller et al., 1983), aortic stenosis, VSD, ASD, and PDA. Caution must be voiced regarding the hypertension in Turner syndrome. Coarctation of the aorta and renal disease or essential hypertension may coexist, and renal disease or essential hypertension may be present in the absence of coarctation of the aorta.

Before scheduling surgical repair of what may appear to be a straightforward coarctation of the aorta, it is prudent to have a renal evaluation and to perform a cardiac catheterization and angiocardiography. The coarctation is usually juxtaductal and the collateral arteries are usually satisfactory. Also, if there is a clear discrepancy between the blood pressures and pulses in the upper and lower extremities, there is usually enough anatomic disease to require resection. However, we have all seen patients who, because of systemic hypertension and a clear pressure and pulse differential, were considered to be certain candidates for surgery, but who proved to have minimal anatomic involvement of the aorta. Conversely, we have seen patients with only borderline hypertension and modest pressure and pulse differentials whose severe anatomic restriction was compensated for and obscured by excellent collateral circulation. We have also seen patients whose elevated systolic blood pressures were unimproved after demonstrably successful coarctectomies, because of the presence of hypertension of other etiology. All of these cases are the exception rather than the rule. The best way to avoid problems in these areas is to be certain that the preoperative evaluation is optimal and that the possibility of confounding variables is shared with the family.

Familial recurrence risk of the 45,X genotype depends on the karyotype. Following a sporadic case, the risk of some form of nondisjunction is 1–2% as in other so-called sporadic cases. Finally, how does the number of X chromosomes influence the type of cardiovascular maldevelopment? Coarctation of the aorta is expressed in males twice as often as in females. Patients with the 45,X genotype are phenotypically female, but lack the full female chromosome complement. One may speculate that the so-called inactivated X chromosome in the 46,XX genotype may produce some gene products that have a modest role in cardiovascular development.

XXXXY Syndrome

One other syndrome of sex chromosomal aberration which has important cardiovascular implications is the XXXXY syndrome. Table 8-13 and Figure 8-13 describe and illustrate some of the features. About 14% have cardiovascular disease (Karsh et al., 1975), and the lesion in almost all

Table 8-13 Features of the XXXXY syndrome

Area	Findings
General	Phenotypic males may have some genital ambiguity, small stature
Neurologic	Retarded, IQ between 25 and 50, moderate hypotonia and joint laxity
Head	Characteristic facies (often confused with mongoloid), low nasal bridge, protruding mandible, occasional flat occiput
Eyes	Epicanthic folds, occasional Brushfield spots, strabismus
Ears	Malformed, low-set
Neck	Short, occasionally webbed
Cardiovascular	Patent ductus arteriosus most common
Extremities	Limited elbow pronation, genu valgum, clinodactyly of the fifth finger
Urogenital	Small penis and testes, frequent cryptorchism
X-ray	Radioulnar stenosis
Dermatoglyphics	Average ridge count is low (< 60), frequent low arches, occasional simian line

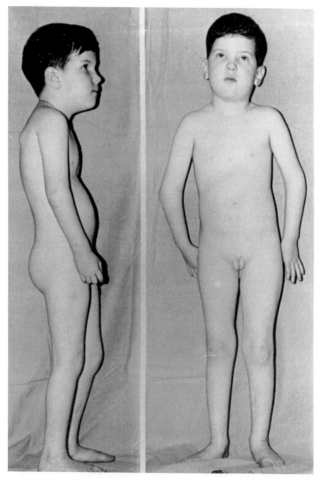

Figure 8-13 This patient with an IQ of 50 has radioulnar synostosis and a small penis which are features of XXXXY syndrome.

cases is PDA. The only other lesions described are ASD and anomalous right coronary artery. The caution here is that just because there is a continuous murmur at the left base does not mean that the patient has a PDA. Fortunately we catheterized our patient (who turned out to have anomalous right coronary artery) and so were prepared to restore a two coronary artery system rather than ligate a PDA.

The interesting etiologic consideration is that these patients with an overabundance of X chromosomes have a malformation (PDA) which is usually expressed twice as frequently in females as in males. As more cases are surveyed, the frequency of PDA decreases so that at 14%, XXXXY syndrome has a relatively low rate of cardiovascular disease when compared with other chromosomal aberrations.

Other Sex Chromosomal Anomalies

Klinefelter (XXY) syndrome has been reported to have an increased risk of mitral valve prolapse. If there is a true increase in risk of structural abnormalities, such as VSD, it is small. The XXX and XXXX aneuploidies do not appear to have an increased risk, and the XXXXX syndrome carries about a 40% risk of cardiovascular abnormalities, most often PDA. Based on the cases reported so far, the XXXYY, XYY, and XXYY anomalies do not have a significant increase in risk of cardiovascular disease.

PERSPECTIVE

In the context of the title of this monograph, the genetics of the chromosomal contribution to congenital heart disease is relatively straightforward. Chromosomal abnormalities produce on the order of 10% of congenital cardiovascular anomalies, essentially always as part of a picture of multiple systems involvement, most of which have been sketched in as defined chromosomal syndromes.

Prevention strategies have progressed substantially in the past decade for combating chromosomal disorders in general, and associated cardiovascular anomalies in particular. Genetic counseling, with indicated family studies, amniocentesis, ultrasound, including fetal echocardiography, and AFP screening are standard weapons in the present armamentarium of prevention.

REFERENCES

Allerdice, P.W., Davis, J.G., Miller, O.J. (1969). *Am. J. Hum. Genet.* **21,** 499.

Baird, P.A., and Sadovnick, A.D. (1987). *J. Pediatr.* **110,** 849.

Berg, W.R., Steele, M.W., and Miller, O.J. (1970). *J. Pediatr.* **77,** 782.

Fineman, R.M., Ablow, R.C., and Howard, R.O. (1975). *Pediatrics.* **56,** 762.

Freedom, R.M., and Gerald P.S. (1973). *Am. J. Dis. Child.* **12,** 16.

Gustavson, K.H., Hitree, V., and Santesson, B. (1976). *Clin. Genet.* **3,** 135.

Guthrie, R.D., Aase, J.M., and Asper, A.C. (1971). *Am. J. Dis. Child.* **122,** 421.

Hodes, M.D., Cole, J., and Palmer, C.G. (1978). *J. Med. Genet.* **15,** 48.

Karsh, R.B., Knapp, R.G., and Nora, J.J. (1975). *Pediatrics.* **56,** 462.

Larco, R.V., Jones, K.L., and Benirschke, K. (1988). *Pediatrics.* **81,** 445.

Lazjuk, G.I., Lurie, I.W., and Ostrowskaja, T.I. (1980). *Clin. Genet.* **18,** 16.

Lemli, L., and Smith, D.W. (1963). *J. Pediatr.* **63,** 577.

Macri, J.N. et al. (1990). *Am. J. Hum. Genet.* **46,** 587.

Matsuoka, R., Misugi, K., and Goto, A. (1983). *Am. J. Med. Genet.* **14,** 657.

Miller, M.J., Geffner, M.E., and Lippe, B.M. (1983). *J. Pediatr.* **102,** 47.

Moerman, P., Fryns, J.P., and Goddeeris, P. (1982). *J Genet Hum.* **30,** 17.

Niebuhr, E. (1978). *Hum. Genet.* **44,** 227.

Niebuhr, E. (1977). *New Chromosomal Syndromes.* Academic Press, New York. p. 273.

Nora, J.J., Torres, F.G., and Sinha, A.K. (1970). *Am. J. Cardiol.* **25,** 639.

Park, S.C., Matthews, R.A., and Zuberbuhler, J.R. (1977). *Am. J. Dis. Child.* **131,** 29.

Rowe, R.D., and Uchida, I.A. (1961). *Am. J. Med.* **31,** 726.

Riccardi, V.M. (1977). *Birth Defects.* **8,** 171.

Rosenfeld, R.G., and Grumbach, M.E. (eds.). (1989). *Turner Syndrome.* Marcel Dekker, Inc., New York.

Schinzel, A., Schmid, W., and Fraccaro, M. (1981). *Hum. Genet.* **57,** 148.

Taylor, A.L. (1968). *J. Med. Genet.* **5,** 227.

Wertelecki, W., and Gerald, P.S. (1971). *J. Pediatr.* **78,** 44.

Wilson, G., Towner, J.W., and Forsman, I. (1979). *Am. J. Med. Genet.* **3,** 155.

Zellweger, H., Ionasescu, V., and Simpson, J. (1976). *Clin. Pediatr.* **15,** 601.

9

Cardiomyopathies and Dysrhythmias

We have chosen to divide our presentation into five major categories of cardiovascular disease. As mentioned in the introduction to this volume, the familial aspects of this broad category, as first ascertained through dysrhythmia were first recognized at the turn of the century (Morquio, 1901; Osler, 1903). Although the majority of these conditions of genetic and epidemiologic interest represent single-gene inheritance, there are notable exceptions, and many of these are optimally discussed in the context of other cardiomyopathies and dysrhythmias. Some of these disorders are characterized by both cardiomyopathy and dysrhythmia, while others may have only one of the two manifestations. Table 9-1 lists selected conditions covered in this chapter and elsewhere in this volume. Certain genetic conditions may have an associated cardiomyopathy or dysrhythmia, but we judge the overall syndrome to warrant the primary attention rather than just the cardiomyopathy or conduction disturbance or both. Of particular interest is the increasing awareness that several myopathies, cardiomyopathies, and dysrhythmias are associated with mitochondrial abnormalities of number and function—and may follow patterns of mitochondrial inheritance (matrilineal) rather than mendelian.

AMYLOIDOSIS III

Of the twenty or more familial forms of amyloidosis, one type, the autosomal dominant amyloidosis III, has significant cardiac manifestations. Although first described in Denmark (Frederiksen et al., 1962), other kindreds have now been reported in the United States and elsewhere (Benson et al., 1987). The features are late-onset (fourth and fifth decades) restrictive cardiomyopathy and congestive heart failure secondary to cardiac amyloidosis. Progression of the disease leads to death over a period of 3–6 years. An absent P wave with a normal QRS complex and failure of atrial depolarization at heart catheterization have been demonstrated in some patients. Husby et al. (1986) have found a substitution of methionine for leucine in position 110 of transthyretin, which plays a role in plasma transport of thyroid hormone.

Table 9-1 Selected cardiomyopathies (CM) and dysrhythmias (DysR) of genetic and epidemiologic interest

Condition	Etiology	Presentation	Discussion
Amyloidosis	A-D[a]	CM, DysR	Chapter 9
Cardiomyopathy, dilated	A-D, A-R[b], M[d]	CM, DysR	Chapter 9
Cardiomyopathy, hypertrophic	A-D	CM, DysR	Chapter 9
Carnitine deficiencies	A-R, ?Mit[e]	CM, DysR	Chapter 9
Conduction disturbances			
Heart blocks	A-D	DysR	Chapter 9
Q-T	A-D, A-R	DysR	Chapter 9
Tachyarrhythmias	A-D, M	DysR	Chapter 9
Endocardial fibroelastosis	M, A-R, X-F[f], ?Mit	CM	Chapter 9
Fabry disease	X-R	CM +[g]	Chapter 6
Friedreich's ataxia	A-R	CM, DysR	Chapter 6
Glycogenoses	A-R	CM	Chapter 6
Kearns-Sayre syndrome	Mit	DysR	Chapter 9
Maternal autoimmune disease	Env[c]	DysR	Chapter 5
Maternal diabetes	Env	CM	Chapter 5
Mucopolysaccharidoses	A-R	CM, DysR +	Chapter 6
Muscular dystrophies	X-R	CM, DysR	Chapter 6
Noonan syndrome	A-D	CM +	Chapter 6
Refsum disease	A-R	DysR	Chapter 6

[a] A-D = autosomal dominant.
[b] A-R = autosomal recessive.
[c] Env = environmental.
[d] M = multifactorial.
[e] Mit = mitochondrial.
[f] X-R = X-linked recessive.
[g] + = other important cardiovascular disease.

CARDIOMYOPATHIES

The three major types of cardiomyopathy are: dilated, hypertrophic, and restrictive. The restrictive form is found in amyloidosis III, glycogen storage disease, scleroderma, and a number of other conditions. Most cases of the restrictive disease, however, do not have primary genetic implications. The other two types of cardiomyopathy are of greater genetic interest and are discussed below.

Dilated Cardiomyopathy

There are several types and several etiologic bases for what eventually results in this form of myocardial disease, including viral pancarditis years earlier, nutritional factors, alcohol, rheumatic damage, and cardiomyopathy as a component of a genetic syndrome. Congestive heart failure, dysrhythmias (heart blocks, atrial fibrillation, supraventricular and ventricular tachycardia), and systemic and pulmonary embolism are common presenting symptoms. The pathologic features are marked ventricular dilatation (predominantly the left) with little to moderate ventricular hypertrophy. The right ventricle has been recognized recently as the site of a cardiomyopathy resulting in sudden death in young people (Thiene et al., 1988).

Familial cases, which represent about one-third of patients, have been reported to follow autosomal dominant, recessive, X-linked, and multifactorial modes (Emanuel et al., 1971; Yamaguchi et al., 1978; Gardner, 1987; Valantine et al., 1989), most often dominant, with 3-, 4-, and 5-generation families. Immunologic factors have been proposed as underlying the disease process in some families which have positive associations with HLA DR4 and B27 and a negative association with DR6Y (Anderson et al., 1984). Whitfield (1961) reported a large family in which both males and females were affected, but the transmission was only through females. Recently heightened awareness concerning myopathies and mitochondrial inheritance should lead investigators to explore such a mechanism in families with matrilineal recurrence of cardiomyopathy.

A number of animal models including those of rats, mice, hamsters, calves, and turkeys have been studied and provide evidence for mendelian, autoimmune, and viral susceptibility modes.

The endstage of dilated cardiomyopathy may be reached by several routes in what is obviously a heterogeneous disease. From the point of view of the genetic counselor, it is necessary to have a thorough genetic-epidemiologic history. If there is clearly direct transmission one must suggest autosomal dominant recurrence risks. If other etiologic factors are apparent, they require careful evaluation.

The clinical course is characterized by progressive to intractable congestive heart failure, dysrhythmias, and sudden death. Symptomatic treatment becomes less effective over time and cardiac transplantation is then a reasonable consideration.

Hypertrophic Cardiomyopathy (HCM)

Idiopathic hypertrophic subaortic stenosis (IHSS), asymmetric septal hypertrophy (ASH), and obstructive cardiomyopathy are among the designations for what appears to be this same disorder, the genetic mode of which was defined as autosomal dominant by Pare and coworkers (1961) and confirmed in extensive studies (Maron and Mulvihill, 1986). Angina, dyspnea, arrhythmias, and syncope are clinical manifestations of the disease, but a frequent and devastating feature is sudden death—generally related to ventricular tachyarrhythmia. The gene for Hypertrophic Cardiomyopathy (HCM) has recently been mapped to 14q1 in the large French Canadian family originally reported by Pare et al. (Jarcho et al., 1989). In a large Italian family, a fragile site on the long arm of chromosome 16 has been found in family members with the disease, but not in those without HCM (Ferraro et al., 1990).

Although invasive studies of a small number of asymptomatic first-degree relatives of affected individuals confirmed that the disease may be present in a mild form, it was echocardiography (echo) that brought a simple noninvasive diagnostic technique to family studies of this disorder (Clark et al., 1973). A septal/left ventricular (LV) wall ratio of greater than 1.3 : 1 was an early criterion for diagnosis by the M-mode echocardiogram of patients with this syndrome. Another M-mode echocardiographic feature is systolic anterior motion of the mitral valve (SAM) as shown in Figure 9-1. The presence or absence of this feature depends on the stage of the disease. SAM may also be occasionally seen in other cardiomyopathies such as those found in infants of diabetic mothers. The myocardial and valvular abnormalities may be appreciated by 2-D echocardiograms and the gradients and anatomy by heart catheterization with contrast angiocardiography (Fig. 9-2).

If one uses echo criteria for the presence of disease, penetrance is close to 100%. On the other hand, severe obstructive disease is much less frequent, on the order of 25%. A polygenic model has also been proposed by Emanuel and Withers, and HLA specificities have been correlated with the disease in different populations (Emanuel and Withers, 1987).

The natural history of the disease varies from the extremes of septal hypertrophy, apparent by echo in the newborn, to ASH developing gradually over many years. We currently advocate periodic echocardiographic

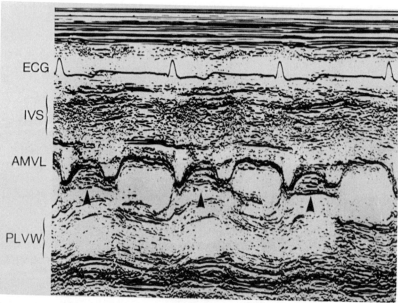

Figure 9-1 M-mode echocardiogram showing greatly increased septal/free wall ratio and septal hypertrophy plus systolic anterior motion of mitral valve (arrow) in hypertrophic cardiomyopathy (idiopathic hypertrophic subaortic stenosis, IHSS).

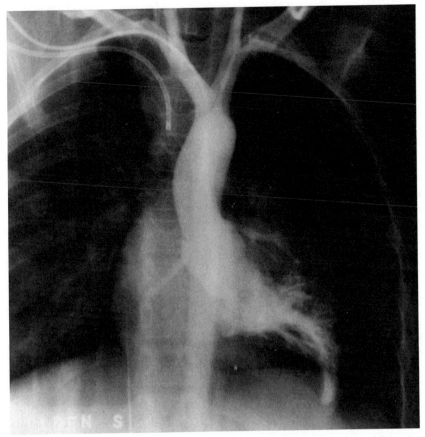

Figure 9-2 Angiocardiogram demonstrating left ventricular chamber obliteration during systole in HCM.

studies (every two or three years) for those family members at risk who are being followed as "normal," so as to be prepared for the appearance of the cardiomyopathy. Those who are asymptomatic, but have ASH indicated by echocardiography, we monitor on more frequent patient-specific schedules with echo.

Unfortunately, sudden death may be the first clue to the presence of the disease. The experience during the past decades was not infrequently repeated in which an attractive high-school student from one of the high-risk families died suddenly without ever having given previous evidence of the disease. This should not happen now if relatives are screened by echo. That is not to say that sudden death will not occur, because this is an ever-present risk (the annual death rate is 2–4%). But the family and physician should be aware of who is at risk, even if asymptomatic. Medical management with beta-adrenergic blocking agents is a first step in management. Maintenance of normal sinus rhythm by the use of various antiarrhythmic drugs, such as amiodarone, and anticoagulation of those who are arrhythmia-prone are often indicated.

Surgical relief may eventually be proposed, but the value of the various approaches has been debated. For those who are symptomatic, there are surgical procedures that may approach either the thickened septum or the septal leaflet of the mitral valve, which balloons into the ventricular outflow tract during the systole (seen as SAM on echo) and is responsible for considerable outflow obstruction.

CARNITINE DEFICIENCIES

Carnitine is a lysine-derived cofactor for fatty acid transport into mitochondria. Primary deficiencies may be systemic or myopathic (Rebouche and Engel, 1983). The more malignant systemic form is characterized by low plasma and tissue carnitine concentration. The myopathic form is characterized by normal plasma levels but reduced muscle carnitine. The systemic form is present in infancy and early childhood with cardiomyopathy, dysrhythmia, skeletal myopathy, hypoglycemia, and encephalopathy. The myopathic form is present in late childhood and in adults as progressive muscle weakness and late cardiorespiratory failure, but without hypoglycemia or encephalopathy. L-carnitine therapy reverses the congestive heart failure and dysrhythmia of systemic carnitine deficiency.

The genetics of the primary deficiency would predictably be autosomal recessive. Indeed, there are substantial data from family studies to support this. Apparently, the systemic and myopathic forms of carnitine deficiency are caused by mutations at separate loci. The systemic form is due to a defect in renal reabsorption. There appears to be considerable genetic heterogeneity among the autosomal recessive forms. Further, the recurrence in some families exceeds expectation for autosomal recessive disease. This, together with the fact that carnitine is involved in mitochondrial metabolic activity, suggests mitochondrial inheritance in some families.

In addition to primary carnitine deficiency, there are several causes of secondary carnitine deficiency including renal, hepatic, and endocrine diseases, pregnancy, valproic acid therapy, and severe malnutrition.

CONDUCTIVE DISTURBANCES

Heart Blocks

Sir William Osler, one of the first physicians to recognize the familial nature of coronary heart disease, was also responsible for one of the earliest reports (Osler, 1903) on familial heart blocks (Stokes-Adams disease). The clinical and electrocardiographic findings in familial cases range

(Gazes, et al., 1965; Michaelsson and Engle, 1972; Barak et al., 1987) from first-degree (prolonged P-R interval), to second-degree (periodic, cyclic, or constant failure of the ventricle to respond to every atrial stimulation), to third-degree (complete atrioventricular block—atria and ventricles beat independently of each other with a slow ventricular rate). From family and twin studies, the atrioventricular conduction time in healthy adults has been suggested to be a heritable trait possibly involving major genes (Møller et al., 1982). Disturbances of conduction from the sinus node to the bundle of His and the fascicles (e.g., right bundle branch block) are among the vulnerable points for blocks and may be found in a single family as expressions of presumably the same genotype. Autosomal dominant inheritance is the rule in familial cases (Waxman et al., 1975). The clinical risk of heart blocks are, of course, syncope and sudden death. Therapy depends on the type and severity of the block, and range from none, to pharmacologic agents, to the need for insertion of a pacemaker.

Q-T Prolongation

Two major genetic syndromes, one with and one without deafness, are associated with a long Q-T interval (see Fig. 9-3), bouts of ventricular tachycardia, and may result in syncope, ventricular fibrillation, and sudden death.

Romano-Ward Syndrome (Prolonged Q-T Without Deafness)
In this autosomal dominant disorder, the Q-T prolongation, which permits extrasystoles to fall in the pathologically prolonged supernormal period of the electrical cycle may be present at rest or in response to exercise.

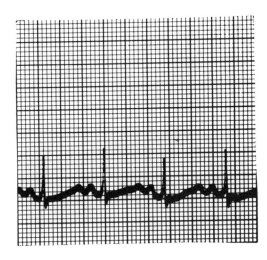

Figure 9-3 Prolonged Q-T interval as seen in patients with Romano-Ward, and Jervell and Lange-Nielsen syndromes.

Historical evidence for the presence of the syndrome in family members may be found by inquiring about fainting spells in childhood. Spells appear to decrease in frequency with increasing age. This is sometimes related to the patient learning to avoid conditions that induce rhythm disturbances, such as vigorous exercise. The electrocardiographic demonstration of the prolonged Q-T interval is diagnostic, but exercise under careful control with the means of cardiac resuscitation at hand may be required to unmask the patient at risk (Fig. 9-4). Because this is an autosomal dominant disease (Ward, 1964; Romano, 1965), cautious electrocardiographic screening is indicated. Beta-adrenergic blockade is the first choice for prevention of dysrhythmic and syncopal episodes (Garza et al., 1970). Sympathectomy may have to be added to the prophylactic regimen of some resistant patients.

Jervell and Lange-Nielsen Syndrome (Prolonged Q-T With Deafness)
This disorder is distinguished from the Romano-Ward syndrome by its mode of inheritance, which is autosomal recessive, and by the additional feature of deafness (Jervell and Lange-Nielsen, 1957). The electrocardiographic findings are identical in the two syndromes and may be present at rest or require exercise to unmask the abnormality. Syncope and sudden death from ventricular fibrillation initiated by extrasystoles falling in the supernormal period represents the identical threat as found in Romano-Ward. The cautions and treatment with beta blockade are the same.

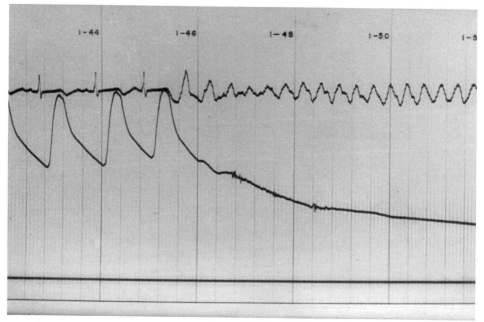

Figure 9-4   Exercise-induced Q-T interval prolongation progressing to ventricular tachyarrhythmia accompanied by severe drop in blood pressure.

Other Tachyarrhythmias

Several other familial tachyarrhythmias are characterized by various abnormalities such as a short P-R interval (the QRS complex may be normal or abnormal with a delta wave and prolongation), atrial tachycardia (usually paroxysmal), or atrial fibrillation, which may be chronic.

Wolff-Parkinson-White (WPW) Syndrome

In the Wolff-Parkinson-White (WPW) syndrome, accessory connections of conducting tissue bypass part or all of the A-V node, and are usually identified by the characteristic electrocardiogram (ECG) abnormalities of short P-R interval and delta wave. Sudden death in ventricular fibrillation triggered by atrial fibrillation occurs in some asymptomatic patients and may be the first manifestation of the disease. Longitudinal follow-up of asymptomatic patients, however, reveals that a considerable number lose the capacity for preexcitation over accessory pathways, which is responsible for their lack of symptomatology and the low mortality in the long term (Klein et al., 1989).

Lown-Ganong-Levine (LGL) Syndrome

The Lown-Ganong-Levine (LGL) syndrome has a short P-R interval and a normal QRS complex. Within these diagnoses, as well as within the entire category of tachyarrhythmias, however, there is a great deal of heterogeneity and variation in the conducting pathways. Familial recurrence of WPW has been frequently reported and within these WPW families there may be patients with LGL.

The genetics of these disorders is not clearly defined as mendelian. There is direct transmission, compatible with autosomal dominant inheritance in reported familial cases, but there is uncertainty as to what the inherited abnormality may actually be.

Treatment includes pharmacologic agents, surgical intervention, and pacemaker implantation. Electrophysiologic studies are being frequently relied on in the selection of appropriate therapeutic modalities.

Endocardial Fibroelastosis (EFE)

This condition, characterized by endomyocardial thickening due to proliferation of collagen and elastin fibers, presents as congestive heart failure, which may respond well to anticongestive measures or progress to early death. Endocardial Fibroelastosis (EFE) does not comfortably fit the expectation for multifactorial inheritance. Autosomal recessive inheritance has been proposed on the basis of some isolated pedigrees, and an X-linked recessive form of the disease is attracting considerable attention (Hodgson et al., 1987). Abnormalities in mitochondria and maternal transmission to male and female offspring suggest possible mitochondrial inheritance in some families. Genomic imprinting may also be a consideration. Mumps virus and Coxsackie virus have also been implicated. Endocardial fibroelastosis has been found to be associated with carnitine deficiency in one family. We still wonder if antiheart antibody may play a role in some cases based on our finding of fluorescent antiheart antibody in the sera of mothers of infants with EFE. The confounding variables are that antiheart antibody increases with increasing parity in mothers, and EFE occurred more frequently in later-born children within the families studied by Chen et al. (1971). It is entirely consistent with available evidence that increasing parity or maternal infection, either of which produces increasing levels of antiheart antibody, may bear a causal relationship to EFE.

A preponderance of females have EFE (M : F 1 : 2). The recurrence risk of 3.8% (Chen et al., 1971) rounds to a counseling figure of 4% for the next sib. This is three times the expectation of recurrence in first-degree relatives under multifactorial inheritance. The concordance for fibroelastosis in subsequent sibs approaches 100%, representing a prominent exception to the experience of ≈50% concordance with most of the structural anomalies. We would recommend using the 4% recurrence risk figure only if there is one sibling with EFE and no other family member suspected of having myocardial disease. In the presence of two affected family members, one should counsel a high mendelian risk, autosomal or X-linked recessive.

Kearns-Sayre Syndrome (Ophthalmoplegia with A-V Block)

This syndrome of ophthalmoplegia, involving pigmentary degeneration of the retina, facial muscle weakness, ptosis, slow neurologic degeneration, and small stature has as its critical feature a progressive atrioventricular block that may change rapidly from unifascicular through bifascicular to complete heart block and sudden death. The important clinical aspect of this problem is recognition of Kearns-Sayre (K-S) syndrome and close cardiologic observation to permit prompt intervention with pacemaker implantation when evidence of progression of the conduction abnormality appears.

The evidence is strong that many familial cases represent mitochondrial inheritance on the basis of transmission being almost exclusively maternal and that the number of affected individuals in sibships significantly exceeds expectation for autosomal dominant inheritance. Deletions in mitochondrial DNA (mtDNA) of skeletal muscle have been identified in the majority of typical cases of K-S (Moraes et al., 1989). Typical K-S syndrome is less commonly found without mtDNA deletions, and ocular myopathy is found in both sporadic and familial cases, with and without deletions of mtDNA. The biochemical defects in K-S syndrome may be related to a lack of translation of mtDNA-encoded respiratory chain polypeptides in some mitochondria, possibly due to a lack of indispensible t-RNAs in these organelles (Nakase et al., 1990).

REFERENCES

Anderson, J.L., Carlquist, J.F., Lutz, J.R., DeWitt, C.W., and Hammond, E.H. (1984). *Am. J. Cardiol.* **53,** 1326.

Barak, M., Herschkowitz, S., Shapiro, I., and Rogiun, N. (1987). *Int. J. Cardiol.* **15,** 231.

Benson, M.D., Wallace, M.R., Tejada, E., Baumann, H., and Page, B. (1987). *Arthritis Rheum.* **30,** 195.

Chen, S.H., Thompson, M.W., and Rose, V. (1971). *J. Pediatr.* **79,** 385.

Clark, C.E., Henry, W.L., and Epstein, S.E. (1973). *N. Engl. J. Med.* **289,** 709.

Emanuel, R., Withers, R., and O'Brien, K. (1971). *Lancet* **II,** 1065.

Emanuel, R., and Withers, R. (1987). In: *Genetics of Cardiovascular Disease.* Pierpont, M.E.M., and Moller, J.H. (eds.). Martinus Nijhoff Publishing, Boston. p. 143.

Ferraro, M., Scarton, G., and Ambrosini, M. (1990). *J. Med. Genet.* **27,** 363.

Frederiksen, T., Gotsche, H., Harboe, N., Kaier, W., and Mellemgaard, K. (1962). *Am. J. Med.* **33,** 328.

Gardner, R.J.M. et al. (1987). *Am. J. Med. Genet.* **27,** 61.

Garza, L.A., Vick, R.L., Nora, J.J., and McNamara, D.G. (1970). *Circulation.* **41,** 39.

Gazes, P.C., Culler, R.M., Taber, E., and Kelly, T.E. (1965). *Circulation.* **32,** 32.

Møller, P., Heiberg, A., and Berg, K. (1982). *Clin. Genet.* **21,** 181.

Hodgson, S., Child, A., and Dyson, M. (1987). *J. Med. Genet.* **24,** 210.

Husby, G., Ranlov, P.J., Sletten, K., and Marhaug, G. (1986). In: *Amyloidosis.* Glenner, G.G. (ed.). Plenum, New York. p. 391.

Jarcho, J.A. et al. (1989). *N. Engl. J. Med.* **321,** 1372.

Jervell, A., and Lange-Nielsen, F. (1957). *Am. Heart J.* **54,** 59.

Klein, G.J., Yee, R., and Sharma, A.D. (1989). *N. Engl. J. Med.* **320.** 1230.

Maron, B.J., and Mulvihill, J.J. (1986). *Ann. Intern. Med.* **105,** 610.

Michaelsson, M., and Engle, M.E. (1972). *Cardiovasc. Clin.* **4,** 85.

Moraes, C.T. et al. (1989). *N. Engl. J. Med.* **320,** 1293.

Morquio, L. (1901). *Arch. Med. Enfants.* **4,** 467.

Nakase, H. et al. (1990). *Am. J. Hum. Genet.* **46,** 418.

Osler, W. (1903). *Lancet* **II,** 516.

Pare, J.A.P., Fraser, R.G., Pirozynski, W.J., Shanks, J.A., Stubington, D. (1961). *Am. J. Med.* **31,** 37.

Rebouche, C.J. , and Engel, A.G. (1983). *Mayo Clin. Proc.* **58,** 533.

Romano, C. (1965). *Lancet* **I,** 658.

Theine, G., Nava, A., Corrado, D., Rossi, L., and Pennelli, N. (1988). *N. Engl. J. Med.* **318,** 129.

Valantine, H.A., Hunt, S.A., Fowler, M.B., et al. (1989). *Am. J. Cardiol.* **63,** 1959.

Ward, O.C. (1964). *J. Irish Med. Assoc.* **54,** 103.

Waxman, M.B., Catching, J.D., and Felderhof, C.H. (1975). *Circulation.* **51,** 226.

Whitfield, A.G.W. (1961). *Quart. J. Med.* **30,** 119.

Yamaguchi, M., Toshima, H., and Yanase, T. (1978). *Jpn. Circ. J.* **42,** 1131.

10
What Will the Future Bring?

The advent of DNA technology makes it reasonable to expect that all or nearly all of the genes involved in genetic predisposition to coronary artery disease (CAD) will be identified in the foreseeable future. The candidate gene approach is likely to succeed provided that all the candidate genes, with respect to CAD risk (see Chapter 1), are examined. It is also likely that the variability gene concept will turn out to be clinically important and that it will be proven that a person's genetic risk for CAD results from the *combination* of level genes and variability genes, with respect to CAD risk factors. Gene-gene interaction in CAD risk will probably be substantiated and new examples found.

As the effect of different variability genes, as well as the nature of gene-gene interaction becomes understood, a deeper insight into pathogenic mechanisms will probably be gained. In the long run, such increased knowledge is likely to have the potential for improving therapy and disease prevention. It is not unlikely that people with different combinations of genes may require different preventive actions. Thus, preventive efforts tailored to the individual's genotype may become part of future preventive cardiology.

Mass screening for CAD risk on a voluntary basis and with complete data protection is likely to improve disease prevention if followed up by adequate counseling and appropriate intervention. The earlier that identification and intervention begin—particularly in childhood—the more successful the outcome should be. A new family-oriented preventive medicine needs to be developed in which the nuclear family would be the target as well as the instrument of implementation (Berg, 1989). It is likely that this approach will improve prevention of CAD and hypertension.

Alternatively, the high-risk strategy of identifying families through a proband with early-onset coronary disease has many advocates. Once more we stress that the child is potentially the subject most likely to benefit from preventive programs such as lifetime commitment to prudent diet, exercise, healthy lifestyle, and avoidance of smoking (Nora, 1989).

Medication may be required for the more resistant hypercholesterolemias, but there are now several drugs available capable of substantially lowering total and LDL cholesterol. The very good news here comes from several studies that demonstrate diminution of plaque size subsequent to lowering of cholesterol levels (Brown et al., 1990). The atherosclerotic process appears to be reversible, even at ages beyond which we previously thought it to be fixed.

In the midst of the composition of good news, a note of concern must be sounded with respect to an emerging and entirely preventable epidemic of early atherosclerosis and coronary events among young people who use anabolic steroids for bodybuilding and athletic enhancement.

Although genes involved in the etiology of other heart conditions such as congenital malformations of the heart should eventually be identified by DNA technology, this may be a more difficult task than to identify genes contributing to CAD risk—except for single-gene syndromes. This is so because of the shortage of good candidate genes for most other heart conditions. It is not unlikely that genetic linkage studies will play an important role in this area. This is a potentially important area of application of progress made in the efforts to map the human genome. Applying hundreds of DNA probes (that in concert define a human genome saturation map) to suitable families would be a formidable task, but could lead to the assignment of genes for several of the more common heart conditions. In the long run this might even make it possible to identify genes of importance for the development of congenital malformations of the heart by "reverse genetics." There will be studies of the functional state of genes contributing to the development of heart malformations or heart diseases. Genetic counseling remains a cornerstone in the prevention of congenital heart diseases (CHD).

Prevention of congenital heart defects caused by chromosomal aberrations also begins with genetic counseling and proceeds through prenatal diagnosis, which is still underutilized, and which includes a host of developing options in addition to amniocentesis.

Identifying and eliminating human teratogens, including those producing CHD has in some instances been highly rewarding, such as in the experience with rubella and thalidomide. For the most part, however, this approach has been disappointing. Problems with traditional epidemiologic studies are reviewed in Chapter 5. Although it must be acknowledged that it is not easy to discover teratogens that cause only a small increase in cardiac defects (particularly common malformations), it must also be pointed out that there have been serious and unnecessary flaws in clinical teratologic studies that invalidate much of the data in the literature. What has made these flaws unnecessary is that guidelines for reasonably accurate teratogen-risk evaluation were determined in the thalidomide investigation over two decades ago. They simply have not been strictly applied. By using the tools we have at the moment, much more can be learned about environmental triggers and how they act on genetically predisposed embryos. Major genes that participate in how the body responds to chemicals should become an even broader investigative area than it is today. It should be technically (if not cost-effectively) possible to screen individuals and families for genetic susceptibility to chemical teratogens.

Since disease risk for several conditions differs with respect to maternal and paternal transmission, not only mitochondrial inheritance, but also the very interesting phenomenon of genomic imprinting must be considered (Hall, 1990). Also, the possibility of gonadal mosaicism in the etiology of disorders with an irregular familial pattern must be entertained and studied (Edwards, 1989). Progress with respect to these genetic phenomena, in studies on cardiovascular disease, could lead to increased understanding of other disorders as well.

At this time it is appropriate not only to look to future developments, but to insist on rigorous application of knowledge and techniques that are already available.

REFERENCES

Berg, K. (1989). *Clin. Genet.* **36,** 299.

Brown, G. et al. (1990). *N. Engl. J. Med.* **323,** 1289.

Edwards, J.H. (1989). *Ann. Hum. Genet.* **53,** 33.

Hall, J. (1990). In: *From Phenotype to Gene in Common Disorders.* Berg, K., Retterstøl, N., and Refsum, S. (eds.). Munksgaard, Copenhagen. pp. 9–36.

Nora, J.J. (1989). *The New Whole Heart Book.* Mid-List Press, Denver.

Index

Page numbers followed by f indicate figures; those followed by a t indicate tables